AD

MW01596284

When I first met Glenn 10 years ago, he told me he was going to beat his chronic lymphocytic leukemia. Since then I have followed his activity and daily regimen, and indeed, he has been extremely successful. Is he an outlier or is his regimen worth studying on a larger scale?

DAVID S. ROSENTHAL, MD
Professor of Medicine, Harvard Medical School
Henry K. Oliver Professor of Hygiene
(Emeritus), Harvard University
Past president, American Cancer Society

A remarkable story of self-efficacy and pure grit. Glenn is a poster child for evidence-based integrative oncology and an exemplar of what might be achieved for others. I highly recommend this book.

MARK HYMAN, MD
Director, Cleveland Clinic Center for
Functional Medicine, and 10-time #1
New York Times bestselling author

n of 1 should be required reading for all cancer patients, but especially anyone who has received a dire prognosis. Glenn's determination, careful research, and willingness to change allowed him to find a cure for his "fatal" cancer, and we all have much to learn from his incredible experience.

KELLY TURNER, PHD
New York Times bestselling author of *Radical Remission:*
Surviving Cancer Against All Odds

I heard Glenn speak at UCSD and was captivated. A special story about resilience and self-efficacy that resonates far and wide!

T. COLIN CAMPBELL, PHD
Bestselling author of *The China Study*
Jacob Gould Schurman Professor Emeritus of
Nutritional Biochemistry, Cornell University

We need to understand that self-induced healing is an entity. It is not a spontaneous remission. We all need to learn from those who don't die when doctors expect them to. Glenn's experience and book will help you to understand and to achieve what is involved in survival behavior.

BERNIE SIEGEL, MD
Author of *Love, Medicine & Miracles* and *The Art of Healing*

How do we maintain a rigorous, scientific, yet open mind when it comes to discovery in medicine? In *n of 1*, Glenn Sabin reminds us that every observation is important—to be woven into the rubric of knowledge so that we may heal with collective experience.

DEBU TRIPATHY, MD
Professor and Chair, Department of Breast Medical Oncology
The University of Texas MD Anderson Cancer Center

A riveting account of one man's journey in fighting his cancer successfully with an unconventional approach. Thought-provoking!

GARY DENG, MD, PHD
Medical Director, Integrative Medicine Service
Memorial Sloan Kettering Cancer Center

n of 1 is a little book with a big message on hope, empowerment and self-efficacy. While "cure" is sadly not possible for everyone, participation in one's healing always should be.

DONALD I. ABRAMS, MD
Chief, Hematology-Oncology, Zuckerberg San Francisco
General Hospital, Professor of Clinical Medicine,
University of California, San Francisco
Co-editor of Abrams/Weil *Integrative Oncology*

There is no such thing as a statistical human. Everyone is utterly unique—each of us is an *n* of 1.

JOSEPH PIZZORNO, ND
Co-author of *Encyclopedia of Natural Medicine*
Editor, *Integrative Medicine, A Clinician's Journal*

Glenn Sabin appears to be one of those few remarkable, determined individuals who become sufficiently involved in their self-healing to overcome a medically "incurable" cancer. Medical science needs to shake off its materialistic bias and study this phenomenon seriously, so that "*n* of 1" can become "*n* of many."

ALASTAIR CUNNINGHAM, OC, PHD
Professor Emeritus of Medical Biophysics at University of Toronto
Author of *Can the Mind Heal Cancer?*

Stories like Glenn's help inspire people to get engaged in improving their health and become active participants in the treatment process. It is important to not over interpret an *n* of 1 experience, yet there is much we can learn from these journeys. Confronting cancer using an evidence-based, integrative approach will likely improve quality of life and the odds of long-term survival.

LORENZO COHEN, PHD
Professor and Director, Integrative Medicine Program
The University of Texas MD Anderson Cancer Center

A rare and intimate look into the journey of a young man expected to die, who defied convention to chart his very personal course back to life and vibrant health. Glenn's courageous story is a testimony to the power of nutrition and the power of one person—an *n* of 1—to help transform the way we look at health and disease.

MICHAEL STROKA, JD, MBA, MS, CNS, LDN
President, American Nutrition Association

n of 1 should be required reading by everyone dealing with cancer on any level—whether patient, caregiver, researcher, or policymaker. It has much to teach us about what is possible.

DWIGHT L. MCKEE MD, CNS, ABIHM
Board certified in medical oncology, hematology,
nutrition, integrative and holistic medicine
Co-author of *After Cancer Care*

This book is an offering—an offering of hope, of wisdom and of determination. While each one of us is truly a unique composition of experiences and choices, we can, nonetheless learn from one another. Glenn has carefully documented his extraordinary experience of using natural means to eradicate leukemia in a way that provides insight, knowledge, hope and inspiration. This book is both encouraging and illuminating.

LISE ALSCHULER, ND, FABNO
Co-author of *Definitive Guide to Cancer* and
Definitive Guide to Thriving After Cancer

I have consulted countless people affected by advanced cancer at MD Anderson Cancer Center and in Israel. These patients all have a common denominator: they all are looking for hope. They would like to meet those few exceptional patients who beat the odds and survived against their doctor's predictions. From my extensive research on exceptional cancer patients around the world, I know that patients need to be active in their decision-making in order to survive. Glenn's story emphasizes this point and should motivate every person affected by cancer to see himself as an *n* of 1. Glenn's approach provides hope, inspiration and motivation to build a proactive plan that can lead to more exceptional patients.

MOSHE FRENKEL, MD
Clinical Associate Professor, University of Texas Medical Branch
Founder, The Integrative Medicine Clinic, The University of Texas
MD Anderson Cancer Center

Glenn's *n of 1* gives us a view into the future of personalized medicine. The patient takes personal responsibility for their health, forms a collaboration team with their doctors, uses longitudinal time series to track the disease and remission, and natural foods and supplements to power the body's immune system to fight off the disease.

LARRY SMARR, PHD
Harry E. Gruber Professor of Computer Science and Engineering
University of California, San Diego
Director, California Institute for
Telecommunications and Information Technology

n of 1 is the amazing tale of Glenn Sabin's resilience in the face of adversity, and is motivation for us all. A moving testament of how a positive attitude plus a healthy lifestyle can have a profound impact on one's life.

NEAL BARNARD, MD
President, Physicians Committee for Responsible Medicine

Glenn Sabin's inspiring story teaches us that it may be possible to reverse even a seemingly incurable disease by becoming proactive in our own care. *n of 1* illustrates the three critical pillars of healing: proper diet, physical activity, and a positive mental outlook—along with personalized nutraceuticals—to establish an anticancer environment that makes healing possible. A must-read for outside the box thinkers and healers alike!

GORDON SAXE, MD, PHD, MPH
Director of Integrative Nutrition
Chair, Krupp Endowed Fund, Center for Integrative Medicine,
University of California, San Diego

Spirited and moving, *n of 1* teaches us so much about hope, resolve, and resilience in the face of cancer.

JUN J. MAO, MD MSCE
Laurance S. Rockefeller Chair in Integrative Medicine
Chief, Integrative Medicine Service
Memorial Sloan Kettering Cancer Center

n of 1

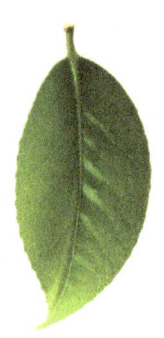

n of 1

One man's Harvard-documented
remission of incurable cancer
using only natural methods

GLENN SABIN

with DAWN LEMANNE, MD, MPH

foreword by
DEAN ORNISH, MD

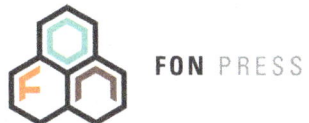

FON PRESS

Published by FON PRESS.

Publisher's Cataloging-in-Publication Data

Names: Sabin, Glenn, author. | Lemanne, Dawn, author. | Ornish, Dean, writer of supplementary textual content.

Title: n of 1: One man's Harvard-documented remission of incurable cancer using only natural methods / by Glenn Sabin, with Dawn Lemanne, MD, MPH; foreword by Dean Ornish, MD.

Other titles: N of One.

Description: First edition. | Silver Spring, MD: FON PRESS, 2016.

Identifiers: LCCN 2016943601 | ISBN 978-0-9975482-0-4 (paperback) ISBN 978-0-9975482-5-9 (paperback special edition) ISBN 978-0-9975482-2-8 (hardcover) | ISBN 978-0-9975482-6-6 (hardcover special edition) | ISBN 978-0-9975482-1-1 (eBook)

Subjects: LCSH: Sabin, Glenn—Health. | Chronic lymphocytic leukemia— Patients—Biography. | Chronic lymphocytic leukemia—Alternative treatment. | Cancer—Patients—Rehabilitation. | Cancer—Psychological aspects. | Self-care, Health. | LCGFT: Autobiographies. | BISAC: BIOGRAPHY & AUTOBIOGRAPHY / Medical | HEALTH & FITNESS / Diseases / Cancer. | BODY, MIND & SPIRIT / Healing / General.

Classification: LCC RC643 .S23 2016 (print) LCC RC643 (ebook) | DDC 616.99/419092—dc23

Edited by Sarah L. Poynton, PhD
Cover Design by Matthew Rippetoe, Sideman Creative LLC
Interior Design by Katie Craig, Stone Pier Productions

For general information:
Contact us at info@glennsabin.com; call us at; 301-384-2476; or write us at FON PRESS; 705 Milshire Court, Silver Spring, MD 20905.

Ordering information:
FON PRESS books may be purchased for educational, business, or sales promotional use. Please contact the Special Markets Department at info@glennsabin.com.

Printed in the United States of America.

To those affected by cancer who, as I do, seek
the empowerment provided by an integrative
approach to healing, and to the courageous
conventional and integrative oncology
clinicians alike, all searching
for the best treatments for cancer.
This book is dedicated to you.

GLENN SABIN

Dedicated to my patients,
who taught me
that we are each an *n* of 1.

DAWN LEMANNE, MD, MPH

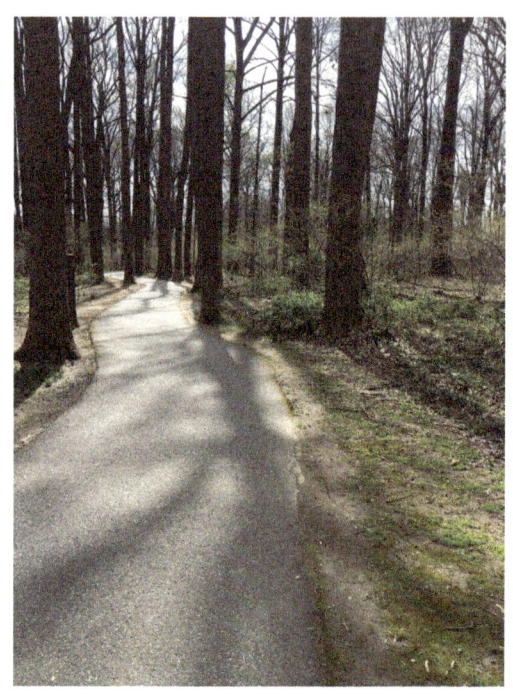

Two roads diverged in a wood, and I—

I took the one less traveled by,

And that has made all the difference.

ROBERT FROST
1874–1963

CONTENTS

DISCLAIMERS

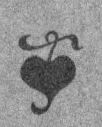

FOREWORD

THIS IS AN EXTRAORDINARY BOOK about one man's journey with cancer and the healing power of comprehensive lifestyle changes.

However, let me say from the beginning that an optimal and responsible approach is to integrate the best of traditional and non-traditional approaches in health and healing, especially with cancer. It would be most unfortunate, even tragic, if readers came away from this book believing that most cancers can be treated with lifestyle changes alone.

Glenn was monitored at every step of the way by a Johns Hopkins oncologist, Dr. Bruce Kressel, a renowned leukemia specialist from the Dana-Farber Cancer Institute at Harvard, Dr. Lee Nadler, as well as a physician with special training in integrative oncology and lifestyle medicine, Dr. Keith Block. They had a clear understanding with Glenn that he would move forward with conventional medical treatments if needed.

It's also worth pointing out that Glenn's cancer—chronic lymphocytic leukemia, or CLL—is usually the least aggressive form of leukemia. More aggressive leukemias, when untreated by conventional means, are almost uniformly fatal within days, weeks, or months. In contrast, 85% of people with Glenn's condition, chronic lymphocytic leukemia, are alive five years after diagnosis. In fact, the course of CLL occasionally extends over decades, although statistically, the average lifespan of those with CLL is shortened. Still, some with CLL, and this includes Glenn, have endured serious illness and hospitalization due to the disease.

Thus, readers who have other forms of leukemia or cancer (which are usually more aggressive) almost always benefit from integrating conventional approaches with lifestyle interventions such as Glenn describes in this book. That CLL comes in many subtypes, some indolent, some aggressive, some intermediate, is increasingly recognized, because of new molecular diagnostic technologies. Using these tests helps physicians determine who might benefit most from new and promising treatments, such as the new targeted immunotherapies.

At the same time that new strides are being made in the conventional treatment of CLL, Glenn Sabin's story is inspiring and illustrates the power of comprehensive lifestyle changes. During the past 40 years, my colleagues and I at the non-profit Preventive Medicine Research Institute, in collaboration with leading medical institutions, have conducted a series of randomized controlled trials and other research studies proving the many benefits of comprehensive lifestyle changes.

These include:

- a whole foods, plant-based diet (naturally low in fat and refined carbohydrates);
- stress management techniques, including yoga and meditation;
- moderate exercise (such as walking); and
- social support and community (love and intimacy).

In our research, we've used high-tech, expensive, state-of-the-art scientific measures to prove the power of these simple, low-tech, and low-cost interventions. These randomized controlled trials and other studies have been published in the leading peer-reviewed medical and scientific journals.

We proved, for the first time, that lifestyle changes alone can reverse the progression of even severe coronary heart disease. There was even more reversal after five years than after one year and 2.5 times fewer cardiac events. We also found that these lifestyle changes can often reverse type 2 diabetes, hypertension, and high cholesterol levels.

My colleagues and I conducted a randomized controlled trial showing that these comprehensive lifestyle changes may slow, stop, or even reverse the progression of early-stage prostate cancer.

Changing lifestyle actually changes the expression of your genes—turning on genes that help keep you healthy, and turning off genes that promote heart disease, prostate cancer, breast cancer, colon cancer, and diabetes—over 500 genes in only three months. Our genes are a predisposition, but our genes are not always our fate.

Our research found that these diet and lifestyle changes may even lengthen telomeres, the ends of your chromosomes that control aging. As your telomeres get longer, your life gets longer, and the risk of premature death from a wide variety of conditions, including many forms of cancer, decreases.

Glenn made many of these lifestyle changes as part of treating his CLL, as well as several supplements described in an open access case report (Cureus 7(12): e441. DOI 10.7759/cureus.441).

He was first diagnosed with CLL at age 28 with an elevated white blood cell count (lymphocytosis), mild anemia, and an enlarged spleen which was surgically removed. Over the next two decades, he suffered two symptomatic leukemia-related events. The first occurred twelve years after diagnosis (at age 40), when he developed fevers, night sweats, and moderate anemia. He was diagnosed with autoimmune hemolytic anemia secondary to his leukemia. He declined conventional therapy in favor of comprehensive lifestyle changes, and recovered from the autoimmune hemolytic anemia though the underlying chronic lymphocytic leukemia remained evident.

Over the second decade following his leukemia diagnosis, he developed abnormally high numbers of white blood cells (lymphocytes) in his bone marrow and then in his blood, with white blood cell counts rising to 55,000/µL (five to ten times normal). In addition to lifestyle changes, he added supplements as described in the open access case report cited above. Over time, his white blood count returned to normal (his doctors would have added conventional treatments had this not occurred). Two years later (at age 48), the peripheral blood and bone marrow were without molecular evidence of chronic lymphocytic leukemia or any malignancy.

In addition to what he did, Glenn took an active role in his recovery and believed in the value of what he was doing—qualities which often enhance healing. At no point did he leave the oversight of conventional physicians. He consulted the medical literature and worked with pre-eminent experts at top cancer centers to get an accurate diagnosis. He was as proactive in undergoing ongoing testing and examinations as he was in implementing comprehensive lifestyle changes. He and his physicians kept up with the current standard of care treatment options and human clinical trials.

Each patient, every person, is truly unique—an "n of 1"—and healing can be different in each case. If you have been diagnosed with cancer or wish to avoid it, please take an active role with your doctors and explore the latest scientific evidence to design a treatment program that is right for you. ❦

DEAN ORNISH, MD
Founder and President, Preventive Medicine Research Institute
Clinical Professor of Medicine, University of California, San Francisco
author, The Spectrum and Dr. Dean Ornish's Program for Reversing Heart Disease
ornish.com

PREFACE

ONE SUMMER AFTERNOON IN 2011, I read a short blog post by Glenn Sabin. Immediately I picked up the phone and called him. The post had mentioned, briefly, his then-partial success using unconventional treatment to hold his chronic lymphocytic leukemia at bay. My purpose in calling was to prove to myself that Glenn's story was too good to be true.

Many times I'd encountered similar reports. These invariably collapsed under slight scrutiny. Usually the patient had a "lump," or a suspicious shadow on an x-ray. But the lump or shadow had never been biopsied, and so the diagnosis of cancer could not be confirmed.

Another common scenario involved someone diagnosed with cancer and treated with conventional therapies known to be effective, but recovery was nevertheless attributed to some non-conventional modality also employed.

To my surprise, Glenn's case was solid. Glenn had documentation of his diagnosis from several respected medical institutions: the National Cancer Institute, Harvard, Johns Hopkins, and George Washington University. He had copies of his pathology and blood test reports. He had letters from his physicians exclaiming surprise at his recovery, despite his refusal of conventional treatment. Glenn's story was the real deal.

That initial phone call lasted two hours. "You're going to write a book about this, aren't you?" I asked him just before hanging up.

"No," Glenn replied. "Too much work."

"But you have to," I said. "The world needs your story."

Glenn balked. So I simply repeated myself, many times. (I am not particularly skilled at persuasion.)

Under my onslaught, he finally acquiesced. But under one condition. We would pair up to get the job done. He would present me with sixty thousand words of recalled conversations and events; I would formulate these into a coherent narrative of his twenty-year struggle with cancer. I would record hours of interviews with Glenn and his wife Linda, and pore over the transcripts. I would interview Glenn's doctors and mentors. Together Glenn and I would organize his huge stack of blood test results, medical records, and biopsy and scan reports. Twenty years' worth.

Glenn is charming and persuasive. Coming from him, the plan sounded straightforward, pleasant even, and I heard myself enthusiastically agreeing. I quickly set aside several hours a day for a thirty-day period to accomplish the task.

That 30-day task lasted four years, during which Glenn endured a major setback to his health. I was honored to be allowed to witness what transpired next. The surprising way Glenn approached that setback—and overcame it beyond anyone's wildest dreams—will forever change how physicians and patients view some cancers. It certainly changed my perspective.

This book is offered with humility. Cancer is a formidable opponent. Not all patients will fare as well as Glenn has, despite all attempts to recover. Furthermore, it's important to point out that the reasons for Glenn's recovery remain unclear.

Glenn is very proactive, and it may very well be that his unconventional treatment program resulted in his recovery. But just as an unknown event triggered Glenn's disease in the first place, might another unknown event have resulted in its remission? An event that had nothing to do with Glenn's actions? After all, association is not causation.

Glenn's story is offered not to answer such questions, but to ask them. Perhaps this book will wedge itself into the cracks in current thinking about cancer and widen them a bit. If so, it will have done its duty.

DAWN LEMANNE, MD, MPH

INTRODUCTION

WHEN I WAS DIAGNOSED with chronic lymphocytic leukemia in 1991, most doctors would have said that modern medicine had no cure.

Most doctors believed then, that finding effective cancer treatments required huge sums of money to be spent on randomized controlled trials, in which expensive pharmaceuticals, many with harsh side effects are tested on numerous human subjects over many years. Such undertakings require the concerted efforts of exquisitely trained, well-funded, and very persistent scientists.

Most doctors believed then that nothing I could do for myself would help me survive leukemia. Although diet, supplements, and exercise—the pursuit of good health—might make my body stronger, my lifestyle choices would have no effect on the leukemia, and would therefore be a waste of time and money.

In 1991, most doctors would have said that there was no way I could successfully treat my own cancer, at home.

It is now 2016, and I am alive. And although I am well, very well indeed, many physicians still say that a patient cannot successfully treat cancer at home.

However, perhaps it can be done. Perhaps I have done it. I don't know. This book is my story, and it is above all the story of an experiment. As an experimenter I have catalogued my failures as well as my successes, in hopes that interested readers might find some instruction in both.

Finally, let me explain how I chose the title of this book, *n of 1*. In an experiment, the number of subjects is represented by the symbol "n." So a typical large clinical trial enrolling a thousand subjects would be described as having an *n* of 1000.

My experiment had only one subject: me. Therefore my study had an *n* of 1. ❧

GLENN SABIN

• PART I •

DEATH SENTENCE

SOMEONE WAS CALLING from the doctor's office to apologize. Would I mind coming in for another blood draw? I didn't mind a bit; I assumed that the samples had been lost or damaged.

It was September 1991, and I was 28. The call from the doctor's office was a great excuse to hop into my '67 Pontiac GTO—my "Goat"—and cruise back to the lab. After giving the blood samples, I didn't give my upcoming checkup a second thought.

A few days later, I woke up charged, ready to blast through the day. The annual checkup barely registered. It was routine maintenance, the last on a long list of errands I planned to check off. How the Redskins would fare that season concerned me more. I kissed my bride Linda goodbye, and hopped into the Goat. With the top down, I roared out of the driveway into a blue and glorious day. We lived in Silver Spring, a Maryland suburb of Washington, D.C., a place where fall is world-class gorgeous. Past verdant lawns I sped, the sun on my face and the wind in my hair. My health status? Simply not on my radar.

I'd skipped breakfast, knowing that somewhere between a haircut and the dentist, I'd snag an oversized convenience-store coffee and a package of pastries, which in those days probably meant something with a decades-long shelf life. Next the Goat would get an oil change. Then came the physical, and if the doc was actually on schedule, I'd be out of there in time to swing by the house, pick up Jazz, our miniature schnauzer, and head for Sligo Creek Park. For an hour, maybe two, my canine buddy and I would amble through the woods, covering as much of the seven-mile trail as we could before getting home in time for dinner.

That was my plan.

My whole life I've made lots of plans, and even as I was driving to my medical appointment, there were many important plans in the works. I probably even had something planned when Linda and I met at a Jewish summer camp when we were 5 and 6 years old, because now she was my wife of two years! I'd always planned to stay close to my family, so Linda and I were remodeling our house, near the neighborhood where I'd grown up. The remodel was stressful, and fraught with the usual delays and cost overruns. But I was proud of the results, a stylish and comfortable home. Exactly as planned. And though we hadn't set any dates, eventually we planned to have children.

I appreciate the finer things in life, so it's lucky I enjoy working hard for a living. I planned to earn enough for a lifestyle that Linda and I could enjoy. In service of that plan, it wasn't unusual for me to put in long days at the media company my father had founded. Shortly after I got married, my father's health had begun to fail, and I found myself running more and more of the operation. I drove myself hard, and I thrived. I loved planning and pushing the business to new heights. Competition stoked me. And the media business let me hang out with musicians, and hear lots of great jazz.

Despite my long workdays, I did not neglect my body. Exercise was planned into my schedule. I worked out almost every day, usually lifting weights. I snuck in occasional unplanned cardio. Exercise was my stress relief, and like my approach to everything, I pushed it. I honestly can't recall being fatigued at that time. I felt like a tank. Indestructible.

So when I showed up at the doctor's office for my "routine maintenance," I expected that last errand of the day to end with a nice slap on the back, and a "See you next year." Instead, the doctor came into the exam room wearing an uncharacteristically solemn expression.

My blood tests showed a problem, he told me. Something serious. Really serious.

So serious, in fact, he had already spoken with my father, whom he'd known for two decades.

It turned out that my original blood samples were not lost or damaged, but abnormal. The doctor had repeated the tests thinking there must have been an error. There was no lab error. The abnormal results were real.

I had a disease, he said. Leukemia. He looked me in the eye. The disease was fatal.

With that news, every plan I had ever made evaporated into thin air. ❦

2

OVER TWENTY-FIVE YEARS HAVE PASSED since that moment in 1991, when I began my cancer journey. I think time has dimmed my memory of that first doctor's appointment, the one that was supposed to be "routine maintenance"; or perhaps what the doctor had to say had always been too difficult to absorb.

I do recall him explaining that I had a blood disorder. It was called chronic lymphocytic leukemia, it was a malignancy, he said, a cancer. Next came something about needing to confirm the diagnosis with a specialist, then a bit of talk about scheduling more tests. Those details are now only a blur in my mind. I vaguely remember stumbling out of the doctor's office and into the lobby. Somewhere I found a payphone. I called home. All Linda could decipher from my incoherent stream of words was that something was very, very wrong. She jumped into her car and sped toward the doctor's office.

Linda found me in the underground parking garage pacing, weeping, beside myself. I slid into the passenger seat of her car, and Linda turned off the engine. Once I'd gathered myself a little, I managed to tell Linda as much as I could fathom of my, of our, predicament.

"I have leukemia. I have to see a specialist. I am going to die."

Linda turned the ignition key, and slowly she maneuvered out of the parking garage. "No," she said. "You're not." ❦

BACK THEN WHAT I DIDN'T KNOW ABOUT LEUKEMIA WAS EPIC. My grandfather had had a strangely named disease called "hairy cell leukemia," and had been treated at the National Institutes of Health. Sadly, he had died from the condition. That all happened before I was born. Other than that bit of family history, my main exposure to the word "leukemia" had been from newspaper and magazine articles, the ones featuring a photo of a cute kid who had lost their hair and needed donations to cover expensive treatments.

I felt sorry for these kids, so I gave what I could. But leukemia, whatever that was, evaporated from my mind immediately afterward.

After my diagnosis, I holed up in my study with books on cancer. What I learned from slogging through the chapters on leukemia was that there is no single disease called "leukemia." In fact, dozens of different blood cancers fall into this category. Each of these leukemia subtypes presents with different signs and symptoms, requires a unique treatment approach, and has a different prognosis.

I also learned that the two major subtypes of leukemia are "acute" and "chronic." Mine was "chronic." At first that reassured me, because "chronic" did not sound as serious as "acute." But as I read, I got some very bad news.

From the textbook descriptions, it was clear that the kids on fund-drive posters usually have one of the acute leukemias. Although "acute" sounded pretty terrifying, I forced myself to read more. What I read was that acute leukemias are the wildfires of oncology, and they can kill within days. The signs and symptoms are anything but subtle: raging fevers, bleeding gums, and deep bruises after the mildest bump. The symptoms bring normal routines to a halt, turning "person" into "patient" almost instantly.

Well, at least "acute leukemia" wasn't me! I felt really healthy and well; in fact, I felt great. Relieved, I kept reading, moving on to the sections on chronic leukemias. What I learned was that chronic leukemias often tiptoe into one's life. At first there may be only a slightly diminished life-spark, a change initially ascribed to laziness, or to waning youth. More often, there are no symptoms at all. The only clue that something is wrong is an abnormal blood test. This was sure sounding like me.

I perked up when I read some good news. With swift and proper treatment, acute leukemias could often be cured. In fact, most children with the disease *were* cured. The procedure that accomplished this was called a bone marrow transplant. Whatever a bone marrow transplant was, it sounded gruesome. But I reminded myself I didn't have acute leukemia. I had the chronic variety. No bone marrow transplants in my future.

. . . .

IN 1991 WHEN I WAS DIAGNOSED, EVERY CASE OF CHRONIC LEUKEMIA WAS FATAL.

. . . .

Relieved, I settled back in my chair and read on.

That was when I came to the bad news. The lack of severe symptoms—at first—doesn't make chronic leukemias a non-problem. Chronic leukemias kill as surely as acute leukemias do. What is different is that in cases of chronic leukemia, death ambles in at a leisurely pace, usually over several years.

Treatment could control some of the symptoms of chronic leukemias. But there was no cure. None. In 1991 when I was diagnosed, every case of chronic leukemia was fatal.

That was what I had: chronic leukemia. Specifically, I had chronic lymphocytic leukemia (CLL): The "always fatal" kind. *I was doomed.* ❦

4

MY FAMILY DOCTOR REFERRED ME TO A HEMATOLOGIST. His name was Dr. Bruce Kressel. When we first met, soon after my annual checkup, his gentle demeanor immediately put me at ease. He examined me thoroughly, noted a subtle swelling in my upper abdomen, and then explained that to confirm the diagnosis of chronic lymphocytic leukemia he would need to do a bone marrow biopsy.

A bone marrow biopsy is considered to be one of the most painful diagnostic procedures. The bone itself cannot be anesthetized, and only the surrounding tissue can be numbed. On an exam table in Dr. Kressel's office, I lay on my stomach and tried to prepare myself. A nurse offered comfort while Dr. Kressel inserted a thick, hollow, needle deep into my hipbone and removed a speck of fatty marrow. It hurt, a lot. But that pain was nothing compared to the agony of the week-long wait for results.

The results were no surprise. My marrow was full of leukemic white blood cells.

It was another gorgeous fall afternoon in Washington, D.C. when Linda, my parents, and I went to Dr. Kressel's office for a long, and very unpleasant, talk. 🌱

5

I WAS SURPRISED TO HEAR that I needed an operation for a blood problem. My predicament, as I understood it then, went something like this:

Healthy bone marrow produces three types of blood cells: red corpuscles, white blood cells, and platelets, all in particular amounts and particular ratios. In contrast, although my marrow was still producing most of its allotment of normal cells, at the same time it was also pumping ten times more cancerous lymphocytes into my bloodstream every day.

Lymphocytes are a subset of white blood cells; they are part of the immune system, and help the body fight infection. But cancerous lymphocytes function poorly, or not at all. Despite this, my marrow insisted on manufacturing these useless cells in such massive amounts, that their sheer number were damaging the rest of my body.

The unceasing production of abnormal cells is a hallmark of cancer. The body makes attempts to control the disease, but when these attempts fail, or are overwhelmed, symptoms occur. In my case, the leukemic cells had lodged in and overwhelmed my spleen.

My spleen was so enlarged Dr. Kressel could easily palpate it, a firm mass distending the upper part of my abdomen. When he pointed this out, initially I was relieved, because I thought I was simply getting fat from Linda's fabulous cooking–despite all my hours at the gym!

The normal spleen hides behind the lower left ribs, far from an examining hand. Its duties include the sequestering of aging or damaged blood cells, dismantling these cells, and sending their building blocks—amino acids, sugars, and fats—back into the bloodstream for recycling.

A healthy spleen weighs only two pounds. Mine weighed seven. It was packed with five pounds of leukemic cells. Not only was my spleen no longer functioning, it was fragile. It could rupture and cause me to bleed to death. Dr. Kressel said it had to come out, and soon.

Once that surgery was done, he said, I might want to consider a bone marrow transplant. I knew nothing about bone marrow transplants. Transplanting anything sounded pretty drastic to me.

I asked if there was any other option. There was. This option was called "watchful waiting." Watchful? Waiting? Waiting for what? Illness? Death? That option sounded even less appealing than a bone marrow transplant! What "watchful waiting" meant was that Dr. Kressel would see me every three months, keeping an eye out for trouble.

What kind of trouble? Patients with CLL typically develop a variety of problems: swollen lymph nodes, anemia, bleeding, blood clots, fevers, infections, or crippling fatigue.

Dr. Kressel explained that when problems eventually arose, I could expect to be treated with chemotherapy or radiation. These treatments would be given in small doses, just enough to ameliorate the symptoms.

Submitting to treatment only when symptoms arose? That sounded good to me, until Dr. Kressel explained that these treatments would not cure me. They would not even prolong my life. All that any such treatment could accomplish was to ease the discomfort the disease caused. That was the most I could look forward to.

By that time, I understood from my own reading what Dr. Kressel was trying to tell me: CLL was incurable. And eventually it was likely to kill me. Had I been a more typical patient, that is, an elderly person, I would likely die of something else before the leukemia got me. But I was young. That meant the disease would have plenty of time to catch up with me. The disease had gotten a huge head start. It already involved my spleen, a complication usually seen only in the last stages of the disease.

My date with death was set. Modern medicine was helpless to postpone it. There was nothing I could do to change this.

Dr. Kressel wrapped up the appointment. We would talk more about treatment another time, after I'd had my spleen removed. Getting that surgery done was urgent.

Mom, Dad, Linda, and I emerged from Dr. Kressel's office into a glorious fall afternoon. I looked at my parent's faces, and saw them filled with despair. I then looked at Linda. What I saw was poise; she was calm and stable. I looked away, towards the beautiful fall colors, blurred now by the tears that filled my eyes. ❦

6

ALTHOUGH WE TRUSTED DR. KRESSEL, Linda was adamant that I not rush into surgery. Splenectomy, as removal of the spleen is called, is a major operation, rife with complications. A 1996 study found that slightly more than half of CLL patients who underwent splenectomy developed problems caused by the operation; some patients even died. What's more, the heavier the spleen, the greater the risk.[1] That statistic should have snagged my attention. With a seven-pounder, I was in high-risk territory.

But I wasn't concerned. I repeatedly pointed out to Linda how young and healthy I was. Except for having leukemia. Linda recognized the difficulty I was having wrapping my brain around my predicament. She felt in her heart this situation was only temporary, but nonetheless, my simplifications—my denial—made me rather useless at decision-making. And yet there were so many decisions to make! So Linda set out, with me in tow, to find a surgeon we could trust with my life. 🌱

---

1 Horowitz J, Smith JL, Weber TK, Rodriguez-Bigas MA, Petrelli NJ. Postoperative complications after splenectomy for hematologic malignancies. Annals of Surgery. 1996;223(3):290-296.

7

IT TOOK US SEVERAL WEEKS to interview three surgeons, all highly respected. We chose the most seasoned. I liked him best because, of the three, he spent the least time listing all the unsettling risks of splenectomy. I needed to concentrate on the positive. The operation was scheduled for the end of November.

And that's how September 1991 came to a close. Football was underway, and for the next two months, I cheered the Redskins through a season that would take them all the way to a Super Bowl win. I also drew up my first will, reviewed my life insurance policies, and reorganized my finances. I wanted to make things as easy as possible for Linda, just in case I didn't survive the splenectomy.

Still, I tried to look on the bright side. That took effort. But I found myself enjoying small things like the autumn chill, and the crunch of leaves underfoot as Jazz and I ambled the trails of Sligo Creek Park. Life seemed precious. And fragile.

I checked into the hospital on Wednesday November 27, 1991, the day before Thanksgiving, as the Redskins barreled toward a playoff spot. To keep my positive frame of mind, I planned what was to come after the operation. Once I had recovered from the splenectomy, I could turn my attention to finding treatment for my chronic lymphocytic leukemia. Real treatment. I wasn't interested in palliative treatment, smoothing out painful bumps on the road to death. My new mantra was "cure." I refused to believe I had an incurable—and fatal—disease. ❧

PART II

LEARNING HOW TO
NAVIGATE FOR MYSELF

8

WHILE I WAS IN THE HOSPITAL, Linda installed a large multi-sectional sofa in our family room. After the operation, lying flat hurt. That meant I couldn't sleep in my own bed. So I spent the entire week, night and day, on that sofa. The room was heavily trafficked, so I'd be near my stereo system, near the kitchen, and best of all, near the TV on which my brother and I were planning to watch the NFL playoffs.

But those first days home after surgery were anything but fun. The incision hurt whenever I stood up, whenever I sat down, whenever I rolled over. I hobbled from sofa to bathroom and back again. Doped up on pain pills, whenever I made it to the sofa I did nothing but doze. Jazz dozed alongside me, our naps interrupted by Linda bringing food, gorgeous, healthy food, food I barely touched.

As the first week turned into the second, the pain eased. I managed with fewer pills. My appetite returned. By the third week I could sleep in my own bed. But something was wrong.

It wasn't physical. Certainly the splenectomy had brutalized me. But the physical pain was a relief in one sense: it had displaced the constant, nagging thoughts of leukemia, thoughts that had come upon me before the surgery, thoughts that would eventually plague me for the next two decades, perhaps for life.

As the incision across my abdomen thickened into scar tissue, as pain lessened its constant grip on my mind, I had to work harder than ever to keep morbid thoughts of leukemia from taking over my mind.

Many years later I can claim some success with controlling depressing ruminations. I am not particularly prone to denial. But I have learned to ponder my diagnosis only when I need to, and always in service of a positive health goal, or when searching for helpful information. But while I was recovering from the splenectomy, my ability to corral my attention was abysmal. I felt imprisoned in a failing body, one with ailing leukemic blood in its veins.

Worse, the whole world was busy reminding me that I had leukemia. Whenever I phoned in to the office, my business associates asked how I was feeling. I could sense their genuine concern. I felt guilty for hating it.

Visits from relatives and friends, fewer now that I was obviously improving, always ended with "Don't do anything strenuous!" Even my brother Jeff constantly warned me to "take it easy." The final straw came when Linda's loving care began to grate on me. I'm not proud of this admission, but I began to snap at her when she brought me a bowl of soup or placed another plate of beautifully prepared food on the coffee table in front of me.

Like most 28-year-old guys, I wasn't prone to extensive introspection. But something very deep in me recoiled at the temptation to allow others to pamper me, or worse, the temptation to pamper myself. On a physical level, I was fed up with resting. I had bowed to the necessities of the splenectomy and its aftermath. I had followed the surgeon's orders, and had dutifully lain around for over three weeks.

Now that I was feeling human again, I itched to think about normal things, to think about something, anything, besides leukemia and death. I desperately needed to be busy. The problem was, there wasn't very much I could still do. I was so weak I actually had to let Linda haul the heavier bags of groceries from the car to the kitchen.

I had lost 35 pounds. The idleness of recovery had made my once-powerful arms and legs thin. My brain, floating in the emptiness of a work-free life, conjured up morbid scenarios about how death would come to me.

I needed to use my mind. I needed to use my body. Specifically, I needed to work out. With weights. Heavy ones. But, that was a problem; a big problem. The doctors had forbidden me to lift anything over 15 pounds for six weeks. But I had a worse problem. Thinking about what I could not do was as bad as thinking about death. So four weeks after my operation, I packed a workout bag, grabbed my car keys, slid into the Goat, and roared off to the gym. ❦

9

IT WAS BAD. By the second set of bench presses, my arms were shaking so hard my spotter yanked the barbell from my hands so I wouldn't drop it on my face.

Had I known then what I know now, I might have done things differently. But in those days I approached my body as though it were a machine. The machine was broken, the gym was my repair shop, and free weights were my tools. Maybe that's not a great metaphor, but at the time it helped me get back into life.

Weight training is my sport; always has been, always will be. As a kid I was self-conscious about my small size. At 12 years old, I successfully nagged my parents for a bench and barbell. But it wasn't until I was 18, and a girl I was crazy about snubbed me, that I got serious about bodybuilding. Then I hit the weights. Hard.

For two years I practically lived at the gym, working out once, sometimes twice, daily. I hung out with competitive body-builders, soaking up technical tips, though I never entered competitions myself.

I learned how to maximally stress muscle tissue to increase bulk, how to alternate muscle groups for fast recovery, how to avoid plateauing by changing up workouts every few weeks, how to "stay hungry" for improvement. My body responded rapidly. Within months my chest was broader, my arms solid and defined. I looked people straight in the eye.

Two years after my "girl problem," not only had my body changed dramatically, many of my self-imposed limitations had fallen away. I was 20 years old when I began to realize what a human could accomplish if they dialed their determination to "high." And they made a good, solid plan.

Now, trying to recover from the splenectomy, I decided to draw on that lesson. My abdomen had just been sliced open and stitched back together. Therefore, when I resumed weight training, it would be good to take it easy.

But once I felt the familiar cold of the barbell in my hands, once I felt the pump of blood surging into muscle, nothing could stop me, not even the possibility of a hernia.

I was so sore after those first workouts I needed several days off just to recover. I began to worry that my plan was utterly stupid.

But my difficulties were temporary. It took only a couple of weeks before I was able to work out consistently. And with that, things took off. My body seemed to heal faster than ever. I gained strength and muscle. Even better, my gloomy thoughts vanished. New ideas arrived in orderly waves, and became plans. My energy level soared. With energy came confidence, and eventually, cockiness.

I was getting well. It was time to find a doctor who could cure me. 🌱

10

A FEW WEEKS AFTER THE SPLENECTOMY, I returned to see Dr. Kressel. When it became clear to him that I was uncomfortable just waiting for the leukemia to act before starting treatment, he suggested I obtain a second opinion. At Harvard University, no less! That recommendation suited me well. Although college rankings had been of no interest to me, even I knew that, when it came to academic endeavors, Harvard topped a slew of "top-10" lists.

Soon I found myself in Boston, being examined by Dr. Lee Nadler. Dr. Nadler is a slender man with a warm manner and a penchant for custom-tailored Italian suits. He is also a world-renowned expert in chronic lymphocytic leukemia. In the years that Dr. Nadler has cared for me, he has become Harvard's Dean for Clinical and Translational Research, and is a leading recipient of research funds from the National Institutes of Health.

I was certain that if anyone could cure me, it would be Dr. Nadler. I let him know I was ready to hear all about the various cures, no matter what the risks. I was strong again and confident, itching to take leukemia to the mat.

I would soon learn that leukemia was way out of my league. In fact, it was way out of Harvard's league too.

It was late 1991, and bone marrow transplant procedures were being tested as a possible treatment for a variety of cancers, from lymphoma to breast cancer. After a thorough review of my case, bone marrow transplantation was what Dr. Nadler offered me. Transplanting anything from one body to another sounded like a bad science fiction movie. I perked up though when Dr. Nadler said transplant might offer a small chance of a cure. However, he was careful to point out that no cure had yet ever been confirmed.

I immediately backed away when he told me that 20 percent of patients who underwent the procedure died. Not of leukemia, but of complications from the bone marrow transplant. I'm no math whiz, but I recognized those odds. They were about the same as Russian roulette.

I told Dr. Nadler to skip to the next curative option. He told me that there was no other curative option. I took a deep breath and looked at Linda. She nodded resolutely.

Dr. Nadler thrust a thick three-ring binder at us. Linda and I opened the daunting tome across our knees. It detailed everything about bone marrow transplantation.

Reading it all would have taken anyone weeks. Even so, we began riffling through it. The binder detailed the mechanics of the procedure itself, the average hospital stay, the sterilization processes required to ward off infection, and a number of expected problems like graft-versus-host disease, hair loss, fevers, fungal sinus invasions, the need for multiple blood transfusions, and how to arrange local lodging for family members.

· ·

IN CONTRAST, THE PREPARATIONS FOR THE TRANS-PLANT WOULD RENDER ME STERILE FOREVER.

· ·

While we waded through this massive missive, Dr. Nadler explained that the leukemic cells were being produced by my bone marrow. Therefore, the only way to get rid of the leukemia forever—to cure the disease—was to utterly destroy every last cell in my bone marrow. Wiping out my marrow would require substantial amounts of chemotherapy and radiation. Because the bone marrow is the source of the immune system, I would be at great risk of dying from infection in the first few weeks and months after the procedure.

But at least any immune problems would be temporary. In contrast, the preparations for the transplant would render me sterile forever. I must have looked confused, because Dr. Nadler paused. He was gentle when he explained that the drugs used to destroy the marrow would also damage the testicles. This would leave me unable to produce sperm, unable to have children. If Linda and I planned to conceive in the future, I would need to bank my sperm before starting the transplant process.

My heart sank. I looked over to Linda. She met my gaze, and in her eyes I saw a clear message: "It's okay, Honey. We'll get through this."

Dr. Nadler was continuing. Once my leukemic marrow had been wiped out, it would have to be replaced with marrow from a healthy donor, in a procedure called allogeneic transplantation. The donor's marrow would be injected into my vein, and would eventually make its way through my bloodstream to my empty bone marrow. There, the donor's marrow cells would settle in and replenish my marrow.

But there were a few catches. Because a perfect match was impossible, my donor's immune cells would recognize my own body as foreign. This was an expected outcome. It even had a name: "graft-versus-host disease," (GVHD). Skin and gut would be especially vulnerable, so I would probably get rashes and liver problems.

There were ways to deal with GVHD. They weren't pretty, either. To keep my new immune system from eating me alive, I would have to take strong immune suppressant medications. Ironically, that would leave me vulnerable to new cancers! The deluge of information made me dizzy.

Dr. Nadler asked if I had any siblings. I had two. Marla and Jeff. That was good, he explained. Donation of bone marrow from a sibling was the best chance for a good match. The chances of one of them matching well enough to be a donor was 50%. But if neither Marla nor Jeff's tissue matched mine, there was another type of transplant, the "autologous" bone marrow transplant. This was a second-best option by all accounts. In the autologous transplant scenario, some of my marrow would be removed, placed in a test tube, and "cleansed" of leukemic cells. The cleansed marrow would be frozen and stored for me while the marrow remaining in my body was destroyed. Said destruction would be carried out by heavy doses of chemotherapy or radiation, just as in the first type of transplant.

With the destruction of my leukemic marrow completed, instead of receiving donor marrow, my own cleansed marrow would be injected into my vein. My cleansed marrow would automatically home in on the empty marrow spaces in my bones, and over the course of a month or two would completely reconstitute my marrow.

The theory behind this, of course, was that the cleansed marrow would no longer contain any leukemic cells. Although neither Dr. Nadler nor anyone else could know it then, the cleansing process did not pan out as well as had been hoped. Patients who lived through the autologous bone marrow transplant procedure died of recurrent leukemia anyway.

Dr. Nadler is a prudent and intelligent physician. He didn't push either transplant option, and was guarded in his predictions about whether they might help me or anyone else. I felt as though I were picking up on his lack of enthusiasm for transplant, so I asked him to proceed to the next option.

To my great disappointment, it was "watchful waiting." Dr. Nadler must have seen my face fall, because he was quick to point out that on the plus side, delaying treatment meant I could take advantage of whatever scientific discoveries lay in the future.

We would later learn that neither of my siblings were suitable donors. That situation took allogeneic transplant off the table. Truth be told, I hadn't been thrilled by the idea anyway. But loss of that option sent me reeling into a week-long depression.

The second bone marrow transplant option was still on the list: using my own "cleansed" marrow as described above, in an autologous transplant. However, it didn't take me long to chuck that idea away. Why go through a risky experimental procedure that had—so far—not worked out for anyone else?

The decision not to try an autologous transplant left "watchful waiting."

I refused that, too.

It was January 1992, and I had no alternative plan. I felt well, but was told I was dying; and I knew I had to do something about it. What that extraordinary "something" might be was beyond my imagination.

As I moved hesitantly into this next phase of my life, I held on to two principles. First, every day was beautiful. Second, I absolutely had to figure out how to stay alive. With those thoughts guiding me, I plunged back into my life.

I worked out with ferocity, adding pounds of hard muscle to my frame. I pulled long days at the office. Evenings, I let Jazz tug me through the woods at Sligo Creek Park. And on weekends, I took Linda on long, delicious dates. We would hop in the Goat and drive an hour to Chesapeake Bay. There we gorged on local blue crab, licking our fingers and laughing.

During those dates, I marveled at my luck at enjoying life with the woman I loved. I marveled at how wonderful "normal" was. Normal was precious. Beyond precious.

Normal lasted seven months. ❧

11

IT WAS A BRIGHT AND WARM SATURDAY EVENING in July, 1992. Our family had gathered in my sister Marla's backyard for a relaxing evening. I was sitting in a lawn chair, chatting and eating barbecue when I felt a pain deep in my abdomen, a pain so sharp it took my breath away. I let out a gasp and bent forward, clutching my stomach. Silence fell over the little gathering. All eyes turned toward me.

I tried to laugh it off. "I must have caught a bug," I joked.

Since my diagnosis nine months before, I had educated myself about CLL. I could tick off a long list of symptoms to watch out for: swollen lymph glands in the neck, armpit or groin, unusual fatigue, fevers, infections, dizziness, various pains, and so forth. In my usual cocky way, I was secretly reassured by the fact that none of those symptoms had managed to catch me. In fact, other than recovering from the splenectomy, I had felt entirely well, until that evening at the barbecue.

Thank God the pain in my abdomen eased after a few seconds. After another minute or two, I was entirely back to normal, and reassured my worried relatives who had gathered around. Then I pushed the incident out of my mind. I filled my plate with food, grabbed a cold beer, and settled back in my lawn chair.

A few minutes later I took another bite of food. Instantly, unimaginable pain gripped my gut. Nausea swept over me. A cold sweat beaded my forehead. My vision dimmed, and I worried that I might faint.

Linda drove me home. We both figured I had eaten something that was off, and that with Linda's good nursing, I would be back to normal by morning. But that night I got worse. Whenever I ate anything, I vomited. The same happened with sips of water. And with each attempt, my gut twisted into agonized knots.

The misery continued into the next morning. By afternoon, an unrelenting vise of pain gripped my insides. Then I realized I could not empty my bowels. Linda pleaded with me to go to the hospital. I refused. I would not even let her call a doctor. I was unwilling to entertain the possibility that the leukemia had come for me at last. An agonized death was preferable to that news. That attitude was all ego.

By evening I could take the agony no more. My ego was no match for the pain. I dragged myself into Linda's car and she squealed down the block. The drive was a nightmare of pain. Linda blasted through red lights, only to brake mid-block so that I could fling open the car door and heave bile onto the curb. And so we lurched toward Sibley Memorial Hospital in D.C., 45 minutes away.

On that trip, how I prayed! I prayed a police car would stop us, that the officer would see my plight and escort us the rest of the way. If only I could get to the hospital! Once there, my nightmare of agony and nausea would finally end.

No police escort materialized. Not only that, but when I arrived at the hospital, the pain did not end. It was only beginning.

. . . .

I WOULD HAVE DONE ANYTHING TO BE RID OF THE PAIN.

. . . .

Once settled in the emergency room, I was denied narcotic pain relievers. I was nearly out of my mind with pain. This was raw agony, and I couldn't understand why the nurses and doctors wouldn't help me. I begged the doctors and nurses for pain medication. The doctors and nurses refused, always professionally, always courteously. I argued. I pleaded. I raged. But I was too ill to do anything more. So I waited. And suffered.

I would later learn that withholding narcotic pain relievers is standard procedure for a patient who comes in with what doctors call an "acute abdomen." This is med-speak for catastrophic conditions involving the bowel, such as perforations, blockages, bleeding, and so forth. If the symptoms of an acute abdomen—nausea, vomiting, and unearthly pain—are masked by pain-relieving medication, the doctor can underestimate the seriousness of the condition. That can delay diagnosis. The patient, pain alleviated, will promptly die.

I could not have known this. And if anyone had explained this to me at the time, I don't recall that I heard it. Perhaps I was too ill to process anything but my horrific pain. But the experience left me with a bad feeling about medical care.

The diagnosis came several hours later. The problem wasn't the leukemia, at least not directly. It was the splenectomy. Healing from the operation had left scar tissue in my abdomen. This is a common occurrence following major abdominal operations. In my case, during the months since the splenectomy, scar tissue had tightened like a rubber band around a segment of my bowel. I would need another operation to release the scar tissue.

The surgeon asked permission to open my abdomen, find the strangled bowel section, and release it by cutting through the constricting scar tissue, like snipping a rubber band tightened around a finger. I signed the consent papers instantly. I had little choice. I would have done anything to be rid of the pain.

I wish I could say that was the end of this episode in my story, that the doctor simply cut through the scar tissue that was strangling a portion of my bowel and discharged me from the hospital a few days later. But things did not go well for me.

A couple of days after the operation, I began shaking with fever and chills. An infection was eating away at my surgical wound. The surgeon had to remove some of the staples to allow the wound to drain. For days I lay in bed with my abdomen flayed open, while a long tube channeled pus from my belly into a plastic bag.

Even all of this did not prevent the most dreaded of surgical complications: sepsis. This is the medical term used when the bacteria or fungi infecting a wound seep into the blood, and from there they circulate through the body. The surgeon tried several antibiotics, one after another, and in various combinations. Nothing seemed to work. I grew desperately ill. Infection specialists were called in. Then came even more antibiotics.

In the end, a specific combination of antibiotics quenched the infection. I would survive.

Twelve days after I arrived at the hospital, I went home, weak, depressed, and with a drain hanging out my still-open wound. Years later I would learn that seven of ten patients without a spleen who developed a severe infection, typically did not survive.[2] I was one of the lucky three. But I was disillusioned.

I had always admired doctors, their decade or more of education, their dedication, their knowledge. But what I had endured during this latest hospitalization had soured my impression of modern medicine.

Within a few months, my reopened abdomen would heal. But the healing process would leave a swollen lumpy track extending from the middle of my breastbone to my navel. Never again would I be comfortable taking off my shirt in public.

I was grateful for the skill of the surgeon who performed my splenectomy, and I understood that complications such as I had had were par for the course, especially with such a serious operation. I was aware that my life had been saved during this latest hospitalization.

---

2 D J Waghorn. Overwhelming infection in asplenic patients: current best practice preventive measures are not being followed. J Clin Pathol 2001;54:214-218 doi:10.1136/jcp.54.3.214

Sure, I had an ugly scar. But at least I could hide it under clothing. Plenty of people with serious medical conditions routinely suffered even more disfigurement than I had. I was grateful to be alive, and grateful to the doctors who did their best to keep me that way.

But I no longer saw medical doctors as an irreproachable source of healing knowledge. And I was beginning to understand that for my leukemia, modern medicine had almost nothing more to offer me. ♥

12

BY THE SUMMER OF 1993, I had cleaned up my diet quite nicely. Gone were the sugar-laden, fat-laced, salt-encrusted, and deeply barbequed, "foods" I had once eaten without a thought.

Each meal presented me with a choice: I could stuff myself with whatever junk food happened to be around, or I could use meals to take some control of my destiny. With each meal came the chance to give my body and mind the highest quality nutrition, the raw material it needed to maintain itself, and my health. I now looked at each meal as an opportunity to advance my body's functioning. At every meal, breakfast, lunch and dinner, I could work my way toward healing.

That frame of mind was what allowed me to leave behind the steak and cheese sandwiches, packaged pastries and French fries. Sure, I missed those things at first. But I was saving my life. Will power wasn't the issue when it came to unhealthy foods. Knowing what *not* to eat was easy. But what *could* I eat? I knew it had something to do with "whole foods," but I had only a vague idea what "whole foods" were. It was Linda who taught me that "whole foods" were just that: whole. Whole foods went from farm to table in one piece.

I also learned what "organic" meant. I caught on when I realized that "organic" was about what was *not* done to food. Organic food was *not* sprayed with pesticides or chemical fertilizers, was *not* mixed with artificial colorings, flavorings and preservatives.

We also avoided food that was warehoused for weeks or years, pre-cooked, irradiated, gassed, boxed, or vacuum-sealed.

Once Linda had taught me what healthy foods were, and once we'd determined to change course, we ran into what is still a major problem for anyone trying to become truly healthy: finding healthy food! Simply getting fresh, organic, whole foods onto our table required major expeditions to farmers' markets, hippie cooperatives, natural food stores and organic grocers.

In contrast, unhealthy food was everywhere. Crackers, cereals, bread, cola, and canned goods streamed out of supermarkets and fast-food restaurants. Office buildings, elementary schools, and even hospitals, boasted vending machines madly dispensing junk. Gas stations sported entire convenience stores bulging with candy, chips, donuts, lunchmeats, hot dogs, and soft drinks. Years of government subsidies supporting factory farming made these mass-produced "foods" cheap.

Eating healthy food wasn't simply a matter of cost, however. In the 1990's, even the most exclusive restaurants commonly served grains and produce sprayed with pesticides, and meat raised on hormones and antibiotics. Fast-forward some 25 years to 2016 and there is increasing demand for real food, not only from individual consumers at home, but also from stores and restaurants. To this day, however, healthy food remains out of reach for many Americans, especially those in poverty-stricken inner city and rural areas.

Linda and I were determined to avoid mass-produced, chemical-laden, non-foods. In those early days, how we struggled to find unsprayed produce! Fortunately, though, nowadays it's easy for Linda and I to find fresh, unsprayed produce at natural foods grocery stores and even some larger chains. And over the years, we've found other sources for healthy food in our area, like farmers' markets. However, we have to be ever vigilant. It requires particular effort to confirm that packaged foods come from respectable companies that take pride in guaranteeing clean, healthy ingredients.

Although my decision to begin watching what I put into my mouth was pretty sudden, the process of perfecting my diet took time. Our choice of vegetables and grains were limited at first. But as we became savvier shoppers, our food palette (pun intended) broadened.

Gradually, kale, spinach, broccoli, carrots, cucumbers, bell peppers, tomatoes, and onions began appearing on my plate, sometimes beside a steaming heap of brown rice. Berries, melons, apples, and pears rounded out our meals, and became the prescription for my lifelong sweet tooth!

Linda soon enrolled in vegan cooking classes. There she learned all about the powerful nutrients found in legumes, sea vegetables, beans, grains, soy, tempeh, and most importantly, in our everyday vegetables.

Linda learned how to decipher the often-impenetrable labels for ingredients on canned and packaged foods. In the past when we used canned foods, we strove for those without added sugar. But once Linda found out that most food cans, even those used by many health-conscious companies, are lined with the carcinogenic plastic BPA, she avoided canned foods. We do now use canned foods, but only from the few companies that use BPA-free cans. Linda also learned that non-stick pans and aluminum cookware can leach chemicals into foods, so can those ubiquitous plastic food storage containers. She replaced our cookware with stainless steel and cast iron, and our plastic containers with glass containers.

Soon cookbooks—vegetarian, vegan, and raw—began to fill our kitchen! I have always had an enormous appetite, and am willing to eat just about anything. When Linda suggested we try almost everything in the books, I was more than game. Going through these recipes one by one sounded like a great adventure!

Even when our boys, Miles and Jared, were young, they thrived on our healthy fare. Now that our sons are teenagers, they do explore other foods when out with their friends. But Linda and I are careful to set a good example at home. And I must say, there is not a lot of complaining going on!

Our whole family loves meatless tacos and veggie Reuben sandwiches. And, hands down, our absolute favorite desert is Linda's pumpkin cheesecake. Or maybe it's her coconut haystacks. Or maybe her lemon sorbet made with avocado and agave nectar. To this day, when I devour the rich, creamy goodness of her pumpkin cheesecake, I'm amazed to think that it contains absolutely no animal products! Linda has been spoiling us with these tasty treats for years. In moderation, of course.

My culinary life was so fantastic, I was certain it could not possibly improve.

Then Linda discovered herbs and spices.

Soon mealtimes were announced by the tantalizing aromas of garlic and turmeric wafting through our house. These little miracles made Linda's already wonderful dishes, taste positively heavenly. I bragged to anyone who would listen, that my wife had become a gourmet cook.

But although I'm sure Linda was glad her dishes made me so happy, she had an ulterior motive, one she freely shared with me. Culinary herbs and spices have a long history of use as folk medicines. Scientists have taken notice, and labs from Texas to Tokyo are studying the anti-cancer actions of the turmeric extract curcumin, among many other herbs.

Before Linda's experimentations, had I even given this type of healthy nutrition much thought, I would have imagined that such light and meatless fare would leave me ravenous. But to my surprise, Linda's carefully planned meals deeply satisfied me. After a few months of true, complete nourishment, even thinking about the greasy, nutrient-depleted fare I used to crave disgusted me. In a complete turnaround, I began to crave the massive salads Linda prepared, and all the home-cooked healthy meals I know to be safe and delicious! Linda's enthusiasm for food as medicine had become mine as well. Eating for health became our new normal, and remains so to this day.

Now I feel vulnerable when traveling, faced with the "food" on offer at airports, convenience stores, and chain supermarkets. Traveling can deprive me of one of my main medicines, namely my fresh, healthy diet. Let me spend a few days on the road, searching in vain to find anything healthy to eat, and I start dreaming of vegetables, tofu, and the other culinary delights of Chef Linda.

. . . .

I WISH I HAD LEARNED, AS A CHILD, HOW TO NOURISH MY BODY.

. . . .

It is generally hard to find restaurants that cater to people with plant-based diets. Happily though, organic and vegetarian-friendly places do exist, such as San Francisco, New York City and Seattle. However, I am optimistic that my traveling food choices will continue to improve, because more and more restaurants and stores are responding to the demand for real, whole foods.

But I have to say that even when I'm home and close to my wife's terrific cooking, I cheat. Not often. But I do cheat. I am human after all, and that means I sometimes crave pizza. And a few times a year I'll enjoy French fries. I'm even known to raise a beer when the Redskins score. And to my dismay, and Linda's, our kids take after their old man. They adore pizza—white flour, cheese and all. Who am I to deprive my kids the joy of Dad devouring (I mean sharing) their pizza?

The vast majority of the time I spend doing the right stuff balances the rare occasions I loosen my restrictions. But I want to emphasize that I tighten those restrictions right up again. Going back to our old way of eating is not an option. When Linda and I nourish ourselves deeply, we notice that we not only feel better, we look better and we function better. That makes our choice easy. Why give up clear minds and supercharged energy levels for "food" that now tastes waxy, salty, or sickeningly sweet?

My diet has evolved over time. It will likely continue to do so, because every day Linda and I learn something new about the science of nutrition. For example, although I still base my diet on whole organic foods, vegetables, beans, fruit, and healthy grains, and although I still eat many raw foods every day, I don't follow a strictly vegan regime. I eat seafood of all kinds, and I make a point to eat plenty of cold water fish packed with the omega-3 fatty acids that are so essential for good health. Salmon and halibut are my favorites. I prefer wild fish, but eat farmed fish if it has been raised without genetically modified feed and antibiotics.

Before closing this chapter, I want to touch on juicing. I don't go on juice fasts, but thanks again to Linda (Yes, indeed you do detect a theme here!), I include juice as part of my daily diet. Long ago Linda discovered that juicing is a stress-free way to get the deep nutrition of fruits and vegetables into me. Although I love green drinks, we still haven't figured out how to get green drinks into our kids. But my lucky sons (and I) happily polish off Linda's amazing fruit "cocktails," alcohol-free, of course!

I wish I had learned, as a child, how to nourish my body. I thank Linda for teaching me, and for teaching our sons this important life lesson.

Now that I had maximized my nutrition under Linda's guidance, I began to wonder if there was even more I could do to take care of my health. 🍷

13

DESPITE THE VAST IMPROVEMENTS in my diet, my blood counts remained abnormal. Not by much, but it was clear I still had chronic lymphocytic leukemia. But I felt entirely well, so Dr. Kressel, my hematologist, recommended "not doing anything."

"Not doing anything" wasn't an option for me.

I had cleaned up my diet, eating vegetables and fruits almost exclusively, avoiding pesticide-sprayed foods, and taking supplements and exercising daily. I explained this new regime to Dr. Kressel, and he heartily encouraged my healthy new lifestyle. However, when I pressed him about the effect of my new way of living on leukemia, Dr. Kressel admitted that he didn't think it was likely to help. There was simply no scientific evidence that lifestyle had any effect on leukemia. I understood that one of Dr. Kressel's duties as a physician was to help me be realistic, to keep any overinflated expectations in check. Though, truth be told, I really wanted Dr. Kressel to be wrong about this.

In my hand, in black and white, were my blood test results. The results were still abnormal. True, time was passing, and the values were no worse than when I was diagnosed. But they were no better, either.

It wasn't that my wonderful new diet wasn't working. It was—in some ways. I looked healthy. I had enormous amounts of energy. But I still had leukemia. What more was there that I could do? Would expanding my search beyond diet help?

14

BACK IN 1992, recovered from the splenectomy and the second surgery to resolve the bowel blockage complication, I was working hard at the media business again. During evenings and weekends I read as widely as I could about various diets, cancer treatments, the medicinal use of supplements, and more. I often loitered in mom-and-pop health food stores, reading various treatises on the wonders of bee pollen, seaweed, or selenium.

As you have heard in previous chapters, soon after my diagnosis I began learning about the benefits of eating whole, unprocessed foods, about going light on animal products. I also started learning about restorative sleep, deep hydration, and physical activity. These ideas were the bright side of the natural health movement.

However, my new explorations also brought me to the darker side of the natural health movement. Behind the whole foods movement, there was a flourishing underground society of health evangelists, many touting "natural" cancer cures. None of these purported cures had passed standardized safety and effectiveness tests. A wiser person than I would have hesitated to enter this shadowy realm without guidance. However, having nothing to lose—or so I thought—I plunged in.

Soon I owned a sizable library of books, pamphlets, and periodicals on shark cartilage, the controversial drug laetrile (illegal in the United States), visualization, coffee enemas, special herbal concoctions, electromagnetic field therapy, ozone colonics, energy medicine, and even odder things. I took to sitting for hours on end at the desk in my home office with Jazz at my feet, trying to make sense of this strange landscape.

Anecdote after anecdote repeated the same basic story: an unfortunate person with a gruesome condition would be sent off to die by "the medical establishment," but was then cured by an herb, a spiritual energy field, supplements, diet, or various combinations of these.

It was not lost on me that these tales always omitted mention of sufferers who failed to benefit from whatever treatment was being proffered. That omission raised big questions. I knew that reputable research always reported the percentage of people who failed to respond to a particular intervention.

I also found it strange that all of these "successful" cancer treatments had no side effects whatsoever. Natural agents, those generally regarded as safe, and without contraindications to other natural agents or drugs, tend to be safer than most pharmaceutical drugs. But absolutely no mention of side effects? Attractive, to be sure. But awfully hard to believe. I needed evidence.

· ·

I TURNED AWAY.
I NEVER WANTED TO SEE ANOTHER
"NATURAL CANCER CURE" BOOK AGAIN.

· ·

The purveyors of these natural cancer cures claimed that they could not convince funders to support investigating these non-patentable treatments. I knew this to be a fair complaint, but I could not buy the next part of their argument. That was the claim that natural cures existed, but were actively suppressed by the "cancer industry," a secretive cabal that protected its huge profits at the cost of human lives. But I have to admit, the repeated claims left me with a niggling doubt, one that for better or worse, kept me reading.

I don't consider myself particularly gullible. Even in my vulnerable state, I knew that what sounds too good to be true—a "natural" cancer cure—usually is.

Rather than letting incomprehensible text go as gibberish, I wrote the authors, or phoned them. When I still failed to get answers I understood, I blamed, not the authors, but my lack of scientific training. I spent huge amounts of time, and money, trying to make sense of what I now know was mostly pseudoscientific schlock.

I would later realize that even the most seasoned physicians and scientific researchers find it daunting to sort through mainstream cancer treatment options. To illustrate the amount of reading material that we're talking about, consider that the results of over a hundred randomized clinical trials are published *every day*. Sorting through only the academically rigorous publications is a huge task.

Today, legitimate results about cancer research are available to anyone via PubMed, an online database of reference citations from the biomedical literature (maintained by the U.S. National Library of Medicine, National Institutes of Health). In addition, to make such technically specialized information useful to the public, such entities as the Mayo Clinic, Johns Hopkins University, WebMD, and Medscape publish summaries of this research on their websites. However, even with the tremendous boon of today's internet, it is often difficult for a non-physician to separate charlatans from those who espouse safe and effective cancer treatments.

Back in the 1990's, early in my journey, searching the internet was not yet part of my daily routine. I had no way of knowing whether the strange treatments I was encountering might be helpful, useless, or even worse, harmful. Although I had used all the tools at my disposal to escape my prison of ignorance, I was still firmly behind bars.

One day in 1995, as I sat at home in my study staring at the growing stack of "natural cancer cure" books, it hit me. The doctors had been right. I *was* wasting my time. I had spent years studying this junk, precious time that I could have spent at work, or with Linda. A pang of loneliness made me stand up to go find her, but then I remembered she had gone to the bookstore. I sat down again with a sigh. Nothing about the books in front of me looked interesting; trying to read more of them was useless.

I began to wonder if I was killing myself with negative thoughts. After all, I had read that "negative thinking" could suppress the immune system, an idea that made sense to me. I sank lower into the quicksand of self-pity.

Then something nudged my shin. Jazz was looking up at me, his brown eyes sparkled with mischief, and wagging the stub of his tail so hard his little body shook. Fifteen minutes later, Jazz was pulling me though through the bright, wintry woods at Sligo Creek Park. The cold air and the exertion scrubbed the gloom from my mind.

It was a weekday, and the park was empty, so I let Jazz off his leash. He trotted from this tree to that, raising a leg at each with the seriousness of a ballerina. He carried out his marking with such dignified purpose that I laughed. Clearly, my boy thought he owned the park. Thanks to Jazz, I felt the sheer joy of being alive.

I pulled into the driveway at dusk. A savory aroma met me as I climbed out of the car. My stomach growled as I entered the kitchen and saw Linda opening the oven door. She told me dinner wouldn't be ready for another 15 minutes. I headed for my study, falling into the habit, hoping to read for a few minutes. But just outside the study door, I halted. All those books only called to my fears. Each one tantalized me with the hope that somewhere, deep within the pages, lay my only chance at a cure. I turned away. I never wanted to see another "natural cancer cure" book again.

That night at dinner, I quietly ate Linda's wonderful cooking and listened to the events of her day. She told me she had found an interesting book, one she really thought I ought to check out. It was on natural cancer cures, she said, and I almost choked—not another one! Luckily I knew enough not to protest. Having been married to Linda for six years, the time was long enough to know that when she gets excited about something, I need to pay attention. ♥

15

LINDA HAD SPENT THE AFTERNOON at the local bookstore, where she had come across a slim volume entitled *Alternatives in Cancer Therapy*. She thumbed through a few pages, felt the book "click," and took it to the cashier.

Linda was unusually animated as she told me about this book. Unlike the dumbed-down books I had been reading, she said this book was erudite. It discussed pros and cons, and didn't whitewash anything. Best of all, it was loaded with reference citations—my long awaited routes into the rigorous scientific and medical literature.

I thanked Linda with feigned enthusiasm. After dinner I added the volume to the mountain of books on my nightstand. Once I'd climbed into bed, the yellow cover of the book caught my eye. In fact, it seemed to be staring at me! I opened the book warily. My plan was to merely scan the table of contents, try not to get too disappointed, and go to sleep.

The title of the book was *Alternatives in Cancer Therapy*; nothing new there. But the subtitle: *The Complete Guide to Non-Traditional Treatments* was a pleasant surprise! I was tired of reading propaganda lauding only one treatment. Comparing various approaches really appealed to me.

Next I turned to the back to read about the author Ross Pelton. He was a registered pharmacist, educated at the University of Wisconsin. He had later become a clinical nutritionist and health educator. What really impressed me was his five years as the administrator of what the book claimed was the largest "holistic" cancer hospital in the world. He was not another uneducated vitamin peddler, writing about enzymes *ad nauseum* who was in reality unable to distinguish an enzyme from an elephant. The guy had been around the block in terms of alternative therapies. That experience was good. Very good. Except for one thing.

Being squarely in the "alternative" camp, Pelton could not have a balanced view of mainstream ideas. Or so I thought. Steeling myself for a blast of vitriol about the evil cancer industry and the oncologists who support it, I turned to the preface of Pelton's book. Instead of vitriol, this is what I read: "The reality is that physicians and researchers on both sides of the fence are genuinely concerned with helping cancer patients. The main difference is that conventional researchers generally look for ways to 'attack cancer,' and those espousing alternatives tend to emphasize the need to improve the health of the patient." I was wrong. The guy was for real. And I was hooked.

Linda shot me an I-told-you-so smile and switched off her light. I rose and took the book to my study. The book's first chapter drew the connection between life-style and cancer; the second chapter touched on the political debates surrounding the field. Most of the main chapters discussed vegetarian and macrobiotic diets, reviewed various therapies such as Gerson therapy and Kelley therapy, discussed the role of single nutrients including vitamin E, selenium, and omega-3 fatty acids, and included a long list of herb-based remedies. The final three chapters discussed the role of mind and emotions in healing.

I finished the book the next day, and sat silently for a while, stunned. Up to that point, I had considered my health plan well-rounded. Turns out I was wrong.

At the time I was eating mainly whole foods and fish. I also took a quality multivitamin, vitamin E, selenium, and vitamin C (rose hips). I assumed that, between my diet and the supplements, I was getting all the nutrients my body required. I knew a bit about the role of antioxidants in counteracting free radicals (oxidative stress), and how certain lifestyle choices like smoking created nutrient depletion. However, Pelton's book had showed me how much more I had to learn.

A few days later I composed a letter to Ross Pelton. I told him how much I enjoyed his book, and I told him a bit about my plight. What I really wanted to do was to speak with him in person. Would he consider giving me a consultation? I worked up my nerve and asked.

Two weeks later I was sitting in Pelton's dining room at his home in San Diego, California, with Linda at my side. Pelton and his wife Taffy treated us to a bowl of fresh whole fruit. Their golden retriever, Ginger, rolled over at my feet, begging for tummy scratches. Ginger seemed to understand that I missed Jazz, and was offering me a dog fix!

This was Linda's first visit to San Diego. We both fell in love with the area, and over the years we would return several times. We loved to rent a convertible and drive for hours along the winding golden coast. The scent of the ocean and the mild clime called to a deep place in both of us, a place that longed for ease. What a spot to retire! 🌺

16

ADOPTING ROSS PELTON'S SUPPLEMENT REGIMEN wasn't as bad as I had thought it would be. Although there were suddenly a lot more pills to take, and I had to take things at different times of the day, I made myself some charts, and eventually figured out how to get everything scheduled. Over just a couple of months, I was up and running with my new supplement regimen. Most of the new supplements I got from my local health foods store. Only a Chinese-made product had to be special ordered.

We installed a reverse osmosis (RO) water filtration unit for the drinking water in our home, and I got another unit for my office. After drinking RO water for only a few days, we were surprised how awful tap water tasted! Had we really been drinking that stuff our whole lives? Now, we can't bring ourselves to down even a single glass!

Our short experience with pure, unadulterated water enabled us to immediately taste and smell the chlorine in the tap water routinely served in restaurants. We no longer wanted to drink the stuff that came out of the tap. We purchased bottled water whenever we went out to eat, or bravely took our own! It sounds odd, I know; but it wasn't snobbery. It was simply that, having tasted the sweetness of real, clean, water, we could no longer stand tap water.

When I learned that much of our daily dose of chlorine and other water pollutants is absorbed through the skin and lungs during showers,[3] I decided to reduce our exposure even further. We splurged on the addition of a whole-house chlorine removal system.

For the next several years I continued with Ross Pelton's nutraceutical recommendations. I also carried on with my own program, drinking big glasses of pure, cleansing water, eating whole foods, and diligently training with weights. What's more, Linda, Jazz and I took frequent power walks in Sligo Creek Park.

Once back home, Linda, Jazz and I would cuddle on the couch to watch television; we were content. One fall day after our walk, we noticed that Jazz was acting a little strangely when we got home. He insisted on lying with his head pressed against Linda's stomach. A few weeks later, we found out Linda was pregnant! Jazz was listening to our baby's heartbeat!

Health, a great wife, a family on the way. I definitely had it all. But I was starting to have doubts about the program Ross Pelton had put me on. 🌿

3 Trabaris M, Laskin JD, Weisel CP. Percutaneous absorption of haloacetonitriles and chloral hydrate and simulated human exposures. J. Appl. Toxicol., 2012; 32: 387–394. doi:10.1002/jat.1657.

17

OUR SON MILES WAS BORN IN 1996. When I held him in my arms, I felt complete, and yet sad. I wanted nothing as much as I wanted to be a husband and a father, and for as long as I possibly could. I didn't want leukemia to cut short the precious time I had with my beautiful new son.

And perhaps fatherhood was what made the questions arise. It was not that I thought Ross Pelton's recommendations were wrong. Not at all, it was just that I wanted to keep looking. Perhaps, just maybe, I was missing out on other resources out there that could help me. So I kept my eyes and ears open, eagerly following developments in nutrition, biology, and cancer treatments.

Linda and I quarreled over this new quest, sometimes heatedly. How could I possibly consider changing paths, she wanted to know, when things were going so well? But I couldn't help it.

I was a father now. I would do anything to see my son grow up. That's what kept me ever on the lookout for new information. Whenever I'd hear about other nutritional pharmacologists who were gaining followings, my antennae would go up.

The search came to a head in the fall of 1998. That was when I came across an article in a local magazine about an unusual pharmacy in Bethesda, Maryland, one that would go on to become one of the most famous "alternative" pharmacies. The pharmacy was *The Apothecary*. 🌱

18

NOT ONLY DID *THE APOTHECARY* sell all manner of herbal products and nutritional supplements, it was a compounding pharmacy. This meant that their in-house pharmacists could hand-prepare a prescription to fit a particular need, such as a personalized combination of medications and supplements, a skin-cream or liquid version of a medication, a dose of a drug not available with off-the-shelf pharmaceuticals, and so forth.

At the epicenter of *The Apothecary* was Dr. Irv Rosenberg. Both pharmacist and nutritionist, Rosenberg was working with scores of patients, many with cancer, and using natural agents to complement their conventional care.

A few days after reading the article, I pulled into the parking lot of *The Apothecary*. Across the street lay the sprawling campus of the National Institutes of Health, the largest medical research institution in the world, with its huge hospitals and glass-walled labs rising from acres of emerald lawn. In contrast, *The Apothecary* was one store in a row of two-story retail establishments. I climbed out of the Goat and headed toward the store.

Had anyone asked why I had come to *The Apothecary* that day, I would have replied that I was there to replenish my supplement supply. The truth was, I was satisfying an immense curiosity, one aroused not only by the article, but by friends and acquaintances I'd pumped for information about Irv Rosenberg. They had nothing but praise for the man and his work.

The store was small, and I wasn't the only one interested in the place. The narrow aisles were filled with people perusing products displayed on floor-to-ceiling shelving. Behind a counter, several pharmacists filled prescriptions for long lines of customers. I wandered around, noting the usual pharmacy offerings: aspirin, laxatives, rubbing alcohol. There too, were the high-quality supplement brands I was familiar with, alongside freshly compounded formulations and herbal products. Every square inch of shelf space was packed with products.

As different as *The Apothecary* was from any other operation I'd seen, the place felt right. I decided I wanted to meet Irv Rosenberg.

On January 20, 1999, I was sitting in a small office lined with supplement-filled shelves. Across a desk sat Irwin Rosenberg. Everyone just called him "Irv." He was a short man with a round face, a gentle demeanor, and a joke always at the ready. He offered to talk about diet and exercise. But I felt I was on track with those; my goal for that meeting was to get a fresh set of eyes on my supplement program.

· ·

"GLENN," HE SAID, "YOU ARE IN THE RIGHT CHURCH, BUT THE WRONG PEW."

· ·

Irv bent his head over the paper I'd handed him. On it I had listed the supplements Ross Pelton had recommended. Irv studied the list thoughtfully for a few moments, then peered over his glasses at me. "Glenn," he said, "you are in the right church, but the wrong pew." I wasn't sure how to take that at first. After all, we were both Jewish!

He explained that there were newer agents available, which would help create a stronger anticancer environment within my body. Irv Rosenberg came up with quite a long protocol, so long that, frankly, it left my head spinning.

And before I list those details, do be warned that this list is not meant to be construed as a treatment for cancer. The next thing I'm about to say sounds harsh, but here goes: using this list, or anything else you read in this book, in lieu of seeking personal guidance from your own medical professional, could cost you your life. Just don't do it. So now that you understand that this program was built for me specifically, that it is therefore unsuitable for anyone else, and that you should work with your own health professional to develop a program that fits your needs, I'll proceed to share with you what Dr. Rosenberg recommended to me, and me alone.

One of Rosenberg's top recommendations for me was a proprietary version of vitamin C, calcium ascorbate with bioflavonoids added to enhance absorption.[4,5]

I was also to take a tablet containing a mixture of four yellow and red plant pigments: carotene, lycopene, lutein, and zeaxanthin.

A third recommendation for me was d-alpha tocopherol, part of the vitamin E family.

Irv also suggested I use a fermented mushroom extract containing "active hexose correlated compound" (AHCC).[6]

---

4 Martí N, Mena P, Cánovas JA, Micol V, Saura D. Vitamin C and the role of citrus juices as functional food. Nat Prod Commun. 2009 May;4(5):677-700.

5 The Institute of Medicine Dietary Reference Intakes for Vitamin C, Vitamin E, Selenium, and Carotenoids. 2000. National Academies Press, Washington DC. https://www.nap.edu/read/9810/chapter/1 (http://bit.ly/2cjw8J3)

6 Ulbricht C, Brigham A, Bryan JK, Catapang M, Chowdary D, Costa D et al. An evidence-based systematic review of active hexose correlated compound (AHCC) by the Natural Standard Research Collaboration. J Diet Suppl. 2013 Sep;10(3):264-308

He also recommended a soy extract called genistein,[7] a vegetable extract called inositol hexaphosphate, and colostrum, an antibody-rich secretion of the bovine mammary gland produced at the time of birth.

An article on selenium published by the U.S. National Institutes of Health opened my eyes to how complex nutritional issues can be. I was surprised to learn that epidemiological studies show that human populations with low selenium levels have an increased risk of many diseases, including cancer. Also, the article pointed out that selenium levels in foods depend on where the food is grown, due to varying selenium levels in the soil. Another interesting piece of information from the article: both deficiency and excess of selenium are harmful. And just to make things even more complicated, different people may need different amounts of selenium for optimum health.[8] So it's truly important that you work with your health care provider to ensure you are getting the selenium you need, but not more than you need.

So there you have Dr. Rosenberg's recommendations for me, for my condition only, and at that particular time. You should not undertake this program, but should consult with your own health care provider for a supplement program tailored to your needs.

As I said, I wasn't ready to make an immediate change. After all, I was doing quite well at the time, and Dr. Kressel and Dr. Nadler, my oncologists, were pleased with my status. Nonetheless, I felt it was time to discuss my supplement protocol with them. ❧

---

7 Nagaraju GP, Zafar SF, El-Rayes BF. Pleiotropic effects of genistein in metabolic, inflammatory, and malignant diseases. Nutr Rev. 2013 Aug;71(8):562-72.
8 National Institutes of Health, Office of Dietary Supplements, Selenium Dietary Supplement Fact Sheet. Available at: https://ods.od.nih.gov/factsheets/Selenium-HealthProfessional/ (http://bit.ly/2d7Srrm)

19

THIS IS A GOOD TIME TO EMPHASIZE that I had not thrown mainstream medicine aside; I never have, and never will. During the years I was experimenting with supplementation and consulting with Ross Pelton and Irv Rosenberg, I saw my local specialist, Dr. Kressel, regularly, often several times a year, for blood tests and examinations. Every few years I returned to Harvard's Dana-Farber Cancer Institute for an exam by Dr. Nadler. Every year or two, I submitted to a painful bone marrow biopsy. This test in particular worried me. Gradually, my bone marrow was filling up with more and more leukemia cells.

Both physicians agreed that because I felt so well, I was not in need of treatment. On the outside, my condition looked stable. From the perspective of conventional medicine, the "watchful waiting" was going swimmingly.

I, however, saw it differently. I wasn't watching. I wasn't waiting. I was doing! I was learning everything I could about caring for my body. More, I was taking action, putting everything I learned into practice. Food. Supplements. Exercise. Clean water. And I was doing it *now*.

In that spirit, I discussed my diet and supplements with each of my oncologists. Both Dr. Kressel and Dr. Nadler were guardedly supportive of my efforts at leading a healthy lifestyle. After all, data were trickling in showing that my type of lifestyle was better than smoking, drinking, and stuffing oneself with soft drinks and packaged pastries. But the oncologists let me know that there was no scientific evidence that supplements, diet, and for that matter, any drastic lifestyle interventions were of any use against leukemia. However, Dr. Nadler noted down in my medical record some of what I was doing.

I came away from these discussions with my oncologists with at least one new fact about supplements. The fact of the matter was this: in choosing between Pelton's pew and Rosenberg's pew, I would be very much on my own.

Oddly, it was Rosenberg's "pew" remark that reinforced my refusal to accept anything on faith. No way was I going to start on his plan without doing my own—extensive—research. In that spirit, I gathered the names of the new products he suggested, and set out to review the available literature on every single one of them. There wasn't much to read. ❧

20

THERE HAD BEEN ALMOST NO RESEARCH on the natural products Irv Rosenberg recommended. I soon found out why. Behind the lack of research into natural products lies our patent process. Natural products cannot be easily patented. However, combine a natural product with other natural products or pharmaceuticals, or develop a new delivery method (perhaps a skin patch or inhaled version of the substance), and add expensive legal assistance, and you may be able to obtain a patent.

It is just this requirement—of time and money—that removes any incentive to test the effectiveness of natural products. Why spend the money to find out whether natural product X works if you can't patent it? What will happen is that a competitor will not only sell product X, but will sell it at a lower price than you can, since they didn't have to invest in research. It's a losing proposition.

It's a bit ironic then that patented pharmaceuticals, including important chemotherapy agents, are often derived from natural sources—algae, fungi, bacteria, plants, and animals. In order to patent these materials, pharmaceutical companies alter them, ostensibly to improve them. The claimed improvements include consistency in dosing, increased effectiveness, and enhanced safety. These are meaningful improvements, to be sure.

However, altering natural products can also lead to decreased effectiveness, unforeseen side effects, or both. Often these adverse effects are not discovered until years after the drug has been released. This delay can obscure the risk-benefit ratio of a particular pharmaceutical.

The research cataloging the risks and benefits of pharmaceuticals makes its way into the world in a strange but interesting form: the several feet of finely printed inserts tucked into boxes of prescription medications.

In contrast, I could find little serious research into the effectiveness of unadulterated natural products. For me, this unfortunate reality meant that checking the claims made by those who purvey supplements was nearly impossible. I was left with no choice but to ask this awful question: who was I willing to trust more at this important juncture? Ross Pelton or Irv Rosenberg?

Precisely because I couldn't check into the supplements that these two pharmacists recommended, I took an alternative approach. I set to work comparing the credentials of Pelton and Rosenberg themselves. 🌱

21

BOTH ROSS PELTON AND IRV ROSENBERG were trained pharmacists. This meant that either of them could do what I could never hope to do: assess a drug's value to me.

A pharmacist understands that a synthetic pharmaceutical, a nutritional supplement, or an herbal product, are all drugs. A pharmacist further understands how a small change to a drug's molecular structure—a carbon atom added here, a hydrogen atom removed there—alters the biological activity of a drug.

In addition, a pharmacist can tell whether a drug taken by mouth crosses the gut wall into the blood, thereby being able to travel throughout the body, or whether it is simply excreted with the stool, without being absorbed. What's more, a pharmacist knows how long a drug will linger in the circulation, whether it is actually taken up by the target organ or cells, or is instead simply "ignored" by the ailing parts of the body, and whether it will interact in harmful or helpful ways with other drugs a patient is taking. Finally, a pharmacist knows whether a drug is removed from circulation by the liver or by the kidneys, by a combination of the two, or via other means, such as perspiration, tears, or exhaled breath.

I appreciated the immense skill a pharmacist must labor to acquire, and I was then and remain now impressed by both Ross Pelton and Irv Rosenberg. But I was more impressed by the central position Irv Rosenberg occupied in the supplement world. *The Apothecary* sold in such high volume that the principals from the largest supplement formulators hustled to Irv Rosenberg's door to exchange opinions, and Irv often attended industry conferences. He was privy to the myriad ways products were hyped, and was therefore in a good position to spot a fraudulent claim. That ability, to me, was gold.

Certainly I was grateful to Ross Pelton for his guidance. But what if, I wondered, what if I had not yet reached the limits of my innate healing potential? What if Irv could access more knowledge?

My gut instincts were clear. Those instincts told me that Irv Rosenberg was the next step along my path to wellness.

Linda's instincts were just as clear. "God is giving you a second chance," she snapped. "How dare you throw it away!" The depth of her feelings about this surprised me. I opened my mouth to quarrel with her. My intuition was important. I was going to follow it.

But I stopped. I had long before learned to listen to my wife. At her urging, I picked up the phone.

I dialed Ross Pelton.

22

ANXIOUS BUT FIRM, I told Ross Pelton how impressed I was with Irv Rosenberg, how I was thinking of switching to his nutraceutical recommendations. It was an uncomfortable moment, to say the least. But the discomfort was mine alone. Ross Pelton was, and remains, one of the most egoless, humble humans I have ever had the honor of interacting with. He responded gently to my announcement, and was his usual warm self. When I asked Ross if he would give me an honest assessment of Irv Rosenberg's suggested protocol, he instantly agreed.

To this day, I am grateful for the priceless gifts of knowledge Pelton bestowed upon me. But I understood that loyalty was not the appropriate way to approach the kind of decision I had to make. I was dealing with a serious diagnosis that was considered terminal. I was fighting for my life. Call it what you will—intuition, an inner voice—something told me it was time to move on.

Ross agreed. Adopting Rosenberg's recommendations was a good move, he said. I should go for it. And the decision did feel right, way deep in my bones.

This was 1999. I could not know that four years later that decision would be put to the test. 🌱

23

I FELT WELL IN 2001, so it surprised me when my local oncologist's surveillance tests revealed a new and ominous trend. The leukemia cells in my blood and bone marrow were increasing in number, Dr. Kressel reported. Although the rise was slow, it was steady. The leukemia was on the move.

Dr. Kressel was concerned, but not alarmed. Because I was still symptom-free, he advised simply following the blood tests and my condition more closely.

I decided to make a special trip to Harvard's Dana-Farber Cancer Institute. I wanted to see what Dr. Nadler thought of this new development, and if he agreed with Dr. Kressel's plan. And so in July of that year, Linda and I boarded an early morning flight to Boston.

No sooner had we settled into our bulkhead seats than my mind rushed ahead to the landing at Logan Airport in Boston, and the hassles that I imagined awaited us there. We'd have to grab a cab to the clinic. Once at the clinic, we'd have to check in with the receptionist, and then slog through a whole morning of scans, x-rays, blood draws, a bone marrow biopsy, and finally a meeting with Dr. Nadler.

I needed to get out of this negative mind frame. To accomplish the tasks of the day I needed to remain reasonably upbeat. Now, I have never been attracted to formal meditation. Over the years, I learned to get out of an emotional funk with vigorous workouts, long walks or swims, or by playing with Miles or Jazz. But none of those things could help me now, stuck as I was in an airplane seat, with an hour of flying time still ahead.

At first I tried to calm myself by reading a magazine I'd picked up in the terminal. When I couldn't concentrate on the words, I reclined my seat, closed my eyes, took deep breaths, and tried to relax. Out of the quiet, a tremendous force suddenly thrust my seat into an upright position. I was so stunned that it took me a moment to realize what had happened. The passenger behind me had driven his feet into the back of my seat. I couldn't believe it. I was dumbfounded. And then a raw anger began to fill me. I turned my head and snapped, "What the hell are you doing?" The man gave me a cold stare. This look I knew well. The man was challenging me. Picking a fight.

I sized him up. He was tall with a medium build. My strength likely outmatched his, despite my much shorter stature. He was about my age, so no youthful advantage for him. If he wanted a fight, I could give him a damn good one. Adrenalin pumped through me, fueling a mighty rage, until I felt a hand on my arm.

Linda. She was pregnant with our second child. I broke away from the man's gaze to look at her. I saw the fear in her eyes, fear that I would do something stupid. I heaved a sigh. I had to allay Linda's fears, to show her I was no longer the hot-headed boy I had once been.

· ·

SO INTENT WAS I ON BASHING HIS FACE IN,
THAT I NEVER SAW THE BYSTANDER
WHO RUSHED ME.

· ·

It took an enormous effort not to look at the man again.

Instead, I reclined my seat. I closed my eyes, took another deep breath, and willed myself to become calm. I understood that it was imperative that I somehow get the calming done quickly, or someone would get hurt. Possibly me.

When I was a youth, trouble had a way of finding me. I was small for my age and other kids underestimated my will to defend myself. Let's say I lost very few fights.

Just before I got married in 1989, I lived in a group house with a few other guys. On a night I was stressing over my business and feeling burned out, the behavior of one of the guys particularly provoked me. He ended up in the hospital with his jaw wired shut.

As for me, I felt ashamed. How had I managed to let what should have been a minor annoyance launch me into an uncontrolled rage? I was lucky the whole thing didn't end up in court. There was one positive outcome.

I also learned a valuable lesson about the price of unbridled anger. Or perhaps I should say that I'd always imagined I'd learned that lesson. I was now being offered a chance to prove it, on that airplane ride to Boston.

Only a moment had passed since the man had shoved my seat. But already my rage was subsiding. I had a plan. The plan was simple, if not exactly easy for me. I would take deep breaths, let my emotions dissipate, and turn my thoughts to my upcoming tests. After all, in another hour or so I would be at Dr. Nadler's clinic. I needed to be ready, mentally and physically. I could not afford to expend one more drop of precious emotional energy on the asshole sitting behind me. I relaxed into my seat and began to draw a deep breath. But before I could finish inhaling, the man jammed his feet into my seatback for a second time, forcing me upright. I saw red. I whirled around. "What the fuck is your problem?" I snarled.

There may have been open seats on the plane. I could have taken the mature, high road, and simply moved. But I was pissed off. No way that I was going to be the one to move. So I reclined again. Within a few seconds I felt something on my hair. The man had placed his newspaper on top of my head. I flung it off. I had had enough.

With my heart racing, enraged, and yet angry at myself for losing control, I somehow acted reasonably. I pushed the call button.

The flight attendant appeared promptly. I explained the problem, but I can't remember exactly what she told the man. But whatever it was, it worked. He left me alone for the rest of the flight.

We landed, and Linda and I snatched our carry-on items and hurried off the plane. Part of me wanted nothing more than to smash my tormentor's teeth in. That was why avoiding him was key, and I have to admit that it took an enormous effort. I only managed by constantly reminding myself that Linda was five months pregnant, that I had a medical condition that required attention, and that the last thing we needed was more drama. With a tremendous act of will, I forced myself to focus on placing one foot in front of the other, on walking out of the airport, on finding a cab, and getting on our way to Dana-Farber.

My riveted focus was working. We were approaching the exit, and the man was nowhere around. Feeling safer, we stopped for a moment to organize our carry-on bags. Even so, I was careful to keep my eyes on my tasks. And just then, the man brushed by.

As he passed, he leaned in and whispered in a deranged sounding tone, "You *had* to call the girl." I did not respond, so he repeated his taunt, his voice dripping with contempt. "*You had to call the girl.*"

I lost it. I dropped my bag. I shoved the man as hard as I could. And then we were brawling, right in the middle of Logan airport. Fists flew. The man head-butted me above my eye. Suddenly blood was everywhere. My blood. But my punches were fast and solid, connecting with his head, his ribs, his gut. I was hurting him. I was relentless. I could have stopped then, victorious, but I escalated.

I took him to the ground.

Now I was on top and pummeling away. So intent was I on bashing his face in, that I never saw the bystander who rushed me. He body checked me so hard that I flew six feet and landed on my elbow. Bone fragments from that landing would cause me pain for months afterwards. By then airport security were dashing toward us, with Massachusetts State Troopers on their heels.

But the fight was over. One of my opponent's eyes was swollen shut. Blood dripped from my head, saturating my denim jacket. Someone handed me a towel to apply pressure to my cut.

The police asked each of us if we wanted to press charges. We both declined. I felt responsible for the whole mess. I had started the physical part of the confrontation. I knew it was wrong. And I had jeopardized the whole visit to Dr. Nadler.

But with the help of the airline, which picked up the cost of the taxi ride to the medical center, and a clean Harvard T-shirt I bought at the airport souvenir shop, we managed to get to the medical center.

With Dr. Nadler's help, I was not only able to get my head sewn up by a plastic surgeon, I managed to fit in all my tests and see him in clinic.

Dr. Nadler concurred with Dr. Kressel that although the leukemia was advancing, I needn't submit to chemotherapy, at least for the time being. Closer surveillance would be enough. That my two physicians agreed reassured me.

Linda and I made it back to the airport that evening for an uneventful return flight to Baltimore.

But Linda was not about to let me call the day a success. "You promised me you would control your anger," she said. I felt horrible. I had let her down. I had let myself down. And that was when I got it. Really got it. Uncontrolled anger can be harmful for anyone. It was especially harmful for me as I dealt with my life-threatening disease.

Over the next weeks the cut on my forehead healed. I stepped up my blood tests with Dr. Kressel. They remained abnormal as usual, but I certainly did not feel sick.

The months passed, and that fall Linda gave birth to our second son Jared. A year passed. Then another. Jared and Miles grew, and I felt happy. I felt well, too, entirely well.

I felt perfectly well one June evening in 2003. I kissed Linda goodnight and switched off the lamp on my nightstand. As I drifted off to sleep, I thanked God for my beautiful wife, my two young sons, and my health.

I woke up the next morning with an intense dimness. 🌿

24

THAT MONDAY MORNING everything seemed slow, distant, draped in shadow. When I complained to Linda about the mild headache I had, she took my temperature. I had a slight fever. I must have caught a cold, we decided, or maybe I had the flu that was going around.

So instead of going to work, I went back to sleep. I spent the entire day in bed, only to awaken that night lying in a puddle of sweat. Yet my teeth were chattering.

Washington, D.C. summers are a non-stop steam bath, a damp heat that rules the day and persists through the night. Sweating through summer was how we lived, and we were used to it. I actually prefer sweating through summer to the bitter cold of winter.

But this sweating was different, way different. Not only were my nightclothes soaked, the sheet beneath me was wringing wet, and so was my pillowcase. I felt anything but overheated. In fact, a bone-deep chill had me shivering violently.

I stripped off my clothes, towel dried, and slipped into fresh pajamas. Immediately I felt better. Then we remade the bed. We turned out the lights to go back to sleep. As I drifted off, I figured that with the breaking of my fever, whatever bug I'd had, was on the way out. By morning I'd be fine. I was certain of it.

But morning dawned with me still feeling drained, headachy, and feverish. I spent a second day in bed. Then a third, and a fourth. And although the days were bad, the nights were hell.

It is probably difficult to impress upon someone who has not experienced or witnessed a true night sweat, how completely drenching they are. Each episode left my nightclothes, sheets and pillowcase wringing wet, making sleep impossible. But since the sweats came at least twice, and often three times, a night, taking a shower and remaking the entire bed after each episode began to wreak havoc on my sleep, and on Linda's as well. By midweek, to get any sleep at all, I had to settle for changing into dry nightclothes and simply covering the soaked bedclothes with dry sheets or towels. By Saturday morning, I was exhausted, and I finally told Linda to take me to the emergency room at D.C.'s Sibley Memorial Hospital. ❧

25

ADMISSION TO SIBLEY MEMORIAL HOSPITAL happened in 2003, 12 years into my diagnosis. I'd learned during those years not to automatically assume that every fever or cold symptom heralded my death from leukemia. Pessimistic assumptions seemed unhealthy to me.

But this illness felt different than anything I had experienced before, and I was really concerned. My symptoms were very close to what I understood the symptoms of CLL to be. Nevertheless, I clung with all my might to the idea that the illness might be something else, specifically hand, foot and mouth disease, a mild viral infection that usually strikes children, and to which I might have been exposed.

Linda and I had joined a gym in Silver Spring, Maryland, near our home. It was a family gym with a terrific weight room, tennis courts, racquetball courts, a pool, various fitness classes, a café, and a fabulous child-care center. We felt comfortable leaving Miles and Jared there for an hour or longer while we worked out, because the staff kept them fully occupied and engaged in healthy activities. We were working out practically every day to justify the additional expense!

During the weeks preceding the onset of my symptoms, hand, foot and mouth disease was circulating in local child-care facilities and schools. The boys seemed fine, but my hope was that perhaps one of them had picked up the virus at school or at the gym, and had transferred it to me.

My fear was this: was the leukemia finally making its big move? 🌱

26

SIBLEY MEMORIAL HOSPITAL is nestled in a green and quiet corner of northwest Washington, D.C., a world away from the inner-city poverty that keeps other D.C. emergency rooms humming. Locals call it "Hotel Sibley," for its location, excellent staff, and superb level of service.

The doctors there ran test after test. These showed that almost half of my red blood cells were gone, destroyed by my own immune system. This immunological destruction of blood, called hemolytic anemia, is a well-known complication of chronic lymphocytic leukemia. But hemolytic anemia can also be caused by infections.

That second possibility brought a team of infectious disease specialists to my bedside. They swabbed my throat, checked my armpits for swollen lymph nodes, and ordered a chest x-ray. When those tests revealed nothing, they sent tube after tube of my blood to the lab. Lab technicians injected my blood into sterile bottles filled with different nutrient media. The idea was that if bacteria were present, they would feed on the medium, multiply, and form colonies big enough to detect. These bacterial colonies could then be subjected to testing with various antibiotics, in hopes of finding one to which they were vulnerable.

Today this process of identifying microbes in the blood, and determining their antibiotic sensitivities takes only hours. But in 2003, this process took several days. Those several days could be the difference between life and death for a patient without a spleen, or a patient with CLL. I had no spleen, *and* I had CLL. Either condition renders one supremely susceptible to serious infections, like the one I'd had the last time I was at Sibley for the surgery to remove the adhesions around my bowel. If I had another infection, I could die. I was in deep trouble.

While the blood cultures "matured" for several days, I was treated with broad-spectrum antibiotics, a cocktail of antibacterial drugs that would kill many of the most likely bacterial invaders.

The whole time I felt horrible—hot, cold, achy, weak, and disoriented. And despite the broad-spectrum antibiotics, I did not get better. 🌿

27

LINDA'S MOM, COOKIE, HAD TAKEN OVER the care of baby Jared and seven-year-old Miles while I was hospitalized. That had freed up some of Linda's time. But I refused to let her stay in my room longer than a couple of hours at a time. Having Linda exhaust herself didn't make any sense to me.

I'd seen too many friends and relatives get run down, emotionally, physically, and nutritionally, while trying to support an ill loved one. I didn't want that to happen to Linda. I knew how many tasks had fallen to her now that I was hospitalized. So I cut her visits short, and encouraged her to exercise, to eat well, and to get some real rest.

On the second day of my hospitalization, I saw Dr. Kressel, who came to see me during his daily rounds. I fought through my misery to give him a nod. Then I got right to the question on everyone's mind. Had the leukemia finally come for me? Although I knew in my heart that he couldn't possibly have the answers I needed, I could not stop myself from asking.

Dr. Kressel was, as always, kind, truthful, and as reassuring as the situation permitted. He was in a serious mood though, as I was pretty sick. He also wanted to know if I was so sick because of the leukemia, or was it a viral infection. After some time with me, Dr. Kressel left. Alone now, I wondered if I were dying. That thought seemed so unreal. Was I really about to leave my wife, my two sons? The physical distress I was feeling was bad enough. The thought that I might be dying, and that none of the doctors would be able to help me, was too horrible to contemplate. I lay quietly for a long time, tears streaming onto the pillowcase.

Later that afternoon the infectious disease team made their rounds. I pushed myself up in bed to hear what they had to say. But, they had no news to report, because the tests were still in process. With nothing much further to tell me, the team marched out.

A few minutes later a phlebotomist entered, pushing a sleek steel cart packed with needles and blood tubes. She was cheerful as she pierced the vein in my arm and filled vial after vial with my dark blood. Her task completed, she too, left.

By now I was feeling really alone and isolated. This circumstance was my own doing. Not only had I sent Linda on her way, I had asked the nurses to turn away relatives, friends, and co-workers. I was hoping to preempt the visitation-induced exhaustion I'd experienced during my previous hospitalization.

Now I was *too* alone. Even television held no appeal. Not only was I physically ill, I was deteriorating emotionally. ❦

28

THERE WAS A WINDOW IN MY ROOM. Through it I could see a blue sky and a few fluffy clouds. Outside waited a perfect July day. And here I was cooped up in a cold, clinical setting, with broad-spectrum antibiotics dripping into my vein. Ill though I was, I desperately needed a change of scenery. A bit of "nature therapy."

I slid my legs over the edge of the bed, stood up, and grabbing the IV pole, I slowly walked to the door of my room. My legs felt a little weak. But since I didn't fall over, I kept going, out into the hospital hallway.

Once I got to the end of the hallway I felt pretty good. I wasn't lightheaded or anything, so I headed back in the other direction to extend the walk. I paced around, walking the halls. After walking for maybe 10 minutes, I had seen everything there was to see in my ward, so I returned to my room and got back in bed.

But I couldn't stay there. I stood up again, but this time I went to the window. I looked down. I could see the manicured grounds surrounding the hospital, traffic flowing along MacArthur Boulevard, and a line of trees across the street. Beyond those trees, but invisible to me, lay the Potomac River.

In fact, out there lay the entire world, and a dose of the world was exactly the medicine I needed. I called the nurse. She arrived promptly, and I told her I needed some fresh air. She crossed her arms, and dutifully explained that the doctors still didn't know what was going on with me, and I was still running a low-grade fever, so an excursion was out of the question.

I felt a pang of remorse, because I had put her in an awkward situation. But my life was at stake, and what I needed at that moment was a dose of outdoors. I asked the nurse to close the door to my room. "Look," I said, "I am not asking for your permission, nor am I discharging myself. Here's the deal: I am leaving the hospital building for 45 minutes, but will stay on the grounds. You did not give me permission, but you know where I am. See you in a bit." And with that, I waited for the nurse to leave, grabbed my sunglasses and IV pole, and headed towards the elevator.

I was wearing street clothes, or more accurately loose workout clothes. I hated the way that wearing hospital clothes evaporated my sense of control. To this day, I never wear a hospital gown, even when getting scans as an outpatient.

I wandered the verdant grounds, exploring, with no particular destination. Eventually I came upon a bench and sat down. The sun on my face and arms felt amazing. Birds chirped on branches above me. Even the suburban cacophony of car horns and trucks rumbling past sounded cheerful, almost musical. The earthy smells and the butterflies flitting around the flowers filled me with joy.

. . . .

IF THE DOCTORS COULDN'T FIGURE OUT WHAT I NEEDED, I WOULD HAVE TO FIGURE IT OUT MYSELF.

. . . .

A new energy flowed into me, and I rose to my feet. Rolling the IV pole ahead of me, I left the hospital grounds. Once I'd made my way to MacArthur Boulevard, I felt a guilty glee. And I felt life flowing through my veins again.

I wanted to live.

I would live. If the doctors couldn't figure out what I needed, I would have to figure it out myself.

After about 30 minutes wandering the neighborhood, I headed back to the hospital. I passed my nurse in the hallway outside my room. She gave me a nod, and a discernible smile. Once back in bed I realized that I was tired, but pleasantly so. I fell into a deep sleep. ❦

29

THE NEXT MORNING the infectious diseases team came around. The blood cultures had remained sterile. That meant that a bacterial infection was not the likely cause of my predicament. However, it was still possible, one of the doctors explained, that I had contracted a virus.

Could it be, I wondered aloud, that I had caught the hand, foot and mouth disease virus that had been circulating in the community? Possibly. But one of the doctors explained that blood culture tests would not reveal a viral infection, because viruses cannot be grown in bacterial culture medium. The team excused themselves and filed out.

I understood that the infectious disease team had done all they could. They had searched for an infection, and had found nothing. The broad-spectrum antibiotics they had prescribed had not helped. The symptoms I was having were not caused by any infection they could detect.

That left leukemia as the culprit. Was the disease finally making a move? I tried not to let my thoughts go in that direction. But after almost a week in the hospital I was still having fevers and night sweats, and my blood test results were still a mess.

Dr. Kressel came in that afternoon, upbeat, bearing cheerful news: I could go home! Then he looked at me with more seriousness. He told me that it appeared that the leukemia *had* made its move, and that meant it would have to be treated. With chemotherapy. I was to come to his office the next day to make the arrangements. 🌱

30

I TRUSTED DR. KRESSEL. He was smart, superbly skilled, and caring. But before I would submit to such a life-changing path as chemotherapy, I needed a second opinion. Dr. Kressel quickly arranged one for me at the renowned Johns Hopkins Hospital in Baltimore, less than an hour's drive away. In early July 2003, Linda and I drove to Baltimore to meet with Dr. Richard Ambinder.

Johns Hopkins frequently sits atop those annual "Best Hospital" lists published by *U.S. News and World Report*. In addition, when I considered that Dr. Ambinder is a world-renowned specialist in chronic lymphocytic leukemia, I knew I was in good hands.

I wasn't disappointed. Dr. Ambinder's team gathered around me, shining lights into my mouth, pressing stethoscopes to my chest, palpating my scarred abdomen, inserting a needle into my elbow crease to fill tube after tube with blood, snapping scans onto light boxes, pointing out this and that detail to each other, murmuring and nodding, and jotting notes in my chart.

At last, with his team hovering behind, Dr. Ambinder sat down with Linda and me. Dr. Ambinder had a thick shock of black hair, a pleasant smile, and a way of getting right to the point. He began with the fact that my red blood cell count was dangerously low, and there was no question about the cause: chronic lymphocytic leukemia. ❦

31

THE TERM "AUTOIMMUNE HEMOLYTIC ANEMIA" came up again, as it had at Sibley. Dr. Ambinder carefully explained what was happening inside me. Auto-immune means, "self-immunity." Hemolytic means, "blood-destroying." Anemia means, "lack of blood."

My immune system had been hijacked by the chronic lymphocytic leukemia. The hijacker had turned my own immune system against my red blood cells. Now reclassified as "enemy," my red blood cells were attacked and destroyed by my own immune cells, the same punishment doled out to bacteria or viruses. This out-of-control immune activation was also behind the fevers and night sweats.

Bone marrow is where blood cells are produced, and, luckily, my marrow was working valiantly to replace the missing red cells, churning out new ones as fast as possible. But there was a danger the rate of destruction could outstrip my marrow's ability to replenish red blood cells. If that happened, Dr. Ambinder explained, I would run out of red blood cells.

Linda asked if there was any chance this autoimmune process might stop on its own. Dr. Ambinder was not of the opinion it would. At least, he had not seen that happen in any previous patient. With the severity of the anemia I was experiencing, and in the face of daily fevers and night sweats, he recommended that I be treated immediately. 🐝

32

AS I SAT LOOKING AT DR. AMBINDER and trying to process what he was telling me, a vivid memory flashed through my mind. Although the calendar on the wall assured me it was 2003, I felt as though I had been transported back in time 12 years, back to 1991, when the leukemia was first diagnosed. I recalled sitting first in Dr. Kressel's office, then in Dr. Nadler's office, while the pros and cons of bone marrow transplantation were lobbed back and forth, like the ball at a tennis match.

Mainly I recalled that bone marrow transplant, although high risk, was the only potential cure for chronic lymphocytic leukemia. I'm not sure what jerked my thoughts back to the present, but I was suddenly back in the present moment, aware that Dr. Ambinder was looking at me, waiting for a response. I assumed he was going to tell me I needed treatment. "So I guess I'll finally have to do the bone marrow transplant," I said.

To say that Dr. Ambinder's response shocked me would be an understatement. There was a long moment of silence. Then he gently explained that bone marrow transplantation was no longer offered to patients with chronic lymphocytic leukemia. Not a single patient had been cured of CLL by bone marrow transplantation.

Linda and I looked at each other. I knew exactly what she was thinking. We had been offered that option back in 1991. Had I undergone the transplant, there was a 1 in 5 chance I might have died; I certainly wouldn't have been cured.

What now dismayed me was that the doctors, the *very best* doctors, had included bone marrow transplant among the "reasonable approaches" back in 1991, and now it was off the books. After such a reversal of recommendations, how were we to trust *any* medical opinion going forward?

Dr. Ambinder explained his proposed plan. First, he said, the hemolytic anemia should be treated with an immune-suppressing drug called prednisone. Then, once the hemolysis was under control, several chemotherapy drugs would be given. Every detail of Dr. Ambinder's plan concurred with Dr. Kressel's advice. Dr. Ambinder concluded the consultation by recommending that I proceed right away with Dr. Kressel's advice.

As Linda and I left Johns Hopkins' Sidney Kimmel Cancer Center, an institution that consistently ranked "among the world's finest cancer treatment centers," we felt anything but reassured. I needed more information.

. . . .

HOW COULD I TRUST ANY MEDICAL ADVICE, WHEN THE LAST ADVICE I'D GOTTEN HAD BEEN SO FAR OFF THE MARK?

. . . .

Once home, I called Dr. Nadler at the Dana-Farber Cancer Institute in Boston. Ostensibly, this call was to make sure he had all the latest details of my current illness. My local oncologist, Dr. Kressel, had always kept Dr. Nadler informed, faithfully mailing and faxing reports to the Boston office.

As I waited for Dr. Nadler to come to the phone, I told myself I just wanted to make sure he had gotten the news. But once I heard Dr. Nadler's reassuring voice, I spilled out my misgivings. How could I trust any medical advice, when the last advice I'd gotten had been so far off the mark? And that included his own advice to consider a bone marrow transplant. ❦

33

LOOKING BACK, I have to say that none of my oncologists had ever pushed bone marrow transplant on me. Back in 1991, when I was first diagnosed, that procedure was truly an unknown. Bone marrow transplant had always been presented as *one* of the options; the doctors had held it out as a possible choice, a way of offering hope when I had few paths to choose from. I knew that. Now though, one of those few paths was gone forever; bone marrow transplant was no longer an option.

I blurted out all of these concerns to Dr. Nadler. I probably sounded hysterical. Dr. Nadler's response was simple and compassionate. I was to come see him, immediately. 🌱

34

DROPPING EVERYTHING TO FLY TO BOSTON to see Dr. Nadler at Dana-Farber was easier said than done. Although it was 2003, three events of the year 2001 clung to me, and especially to Linda, who had not been on a plane since my fistfight in Logan Airport. The fight had been in July 2001; it was quickly followed by the 9/11 terror attacks in New York, Shanksville, Pennsylvania, and Washington, D.C.; and then the birth of our second son, Jared, in November 2001. For Linda, air travel had lost every appeal.

Driving to Boston was fine by me. I actually enjoy screaming down a long stretch of asphalt, just Linda and me and some good music. So we dropped Miles and Jared off at relatives, piled into the Land Cruiser, and set out on a road trip to Dana-Farber. Not a good choice.

Though sick, I insisted on driving part of the way. That meant that I was at the wheel when we were pulled over for speeding. My lame excuse about having cancer and needing to get to the hospital, hundreds of miles away, failed to impress the state trooper. He carefully tore my citation out of his citation pad and passed it through the window to me with a serious, "Drive safely."

The clinic visit wasn't much better. After yet another round of tests, Dr. Nadler came in with a worried look. I was still dangerously anemic, he told me. Other blood test results were equally troubling.

There was at least some good news. The CT scans showed no enlarged lymph nodes, (which, had they been present, would have been a classic sign of CLL). Brash, I pointed out that I had never had enlarged lymph nodes. "Glenn," Dr. Nadler said, "You're heading off a cliff."

I got it. I needed immediate treatment. Dr. Nadler recommended a regimen similar to that advised by Drs. Kressel and Ambinder. Dr. Nadler's regimen used most of the same drugs as the other regimens, and on a similar schedule. Dr. Nadler insisted that the details of treatment weren't as important as getting started with something. I was in line for treatment. There was no other choice.

"I'll think it over," I said, unconvinced. Dr. Nadler looked at me thoughtfully, and then asked what I planned to do instead of chemotherapy. I had no answer. ♥

35

THE TRIP HOME TO MARYLAND WAS ARDUOUS. I was running a 100-degree fever, and felt too ill to take the wheel at all. That left all the driving to Linda, including six hours stuck in a traffic jam outside of New York City. We were both irritable. Wisely, I think, we decided to be silent.

That gave me time to think.

I realized that that moment I had dreaded was finally here. The doctors were unanimous: I needed chemotherapy. Not "curative" chemotherapy, but a palliative Band-Aid to get me out of the danger zone and buy some time.

My mind went into overdrive. Should I trust the doctors? And if so, why? After all, they apparently didn't agree on the details of the treatment. That, however, wasn't surprising. Doctors often have different opinions, especially when they are working at the edges of what's known, like my doctors were. Although the doctors might have disagreed about the details of treatment, there was one point on which they were unanimous: treatment wouldn't cure me.

Back then, in 1991, no known treatment could reliably prolong a CLL patient's life. My doctors were the best, but what if their proposed treatment went wrong and I got sicker? What if I died?

As it was, I was hardly living. I was sick with fevers, night sweats, and a miserable flu-like feeling *all* the time. At least the proposed treatment promised to relieve those symptoms.

I reviewed my predicament. CLL was considered terminal. Though some people lived for a number of years with this disease, there was no cure.

What good was treatment, if I was going to die of CLL at an appointed time, and all the king's horses and all the king's men couldn't postpone my day of doom?

It turns out that my present, miserable state contained the answer to that question.

Several months of treatment would almost certainly relieve the horrible fevers, night sweats, and fatigue. And maybe I'd be one of the lucky ones who had a long period of remission after treatment, maybe several years of feeling healthy, or at least feeling better than I was currently feeling.

I was pretty close to deciding to take the chemo, almost ready to wade through the side effects of the drugs, including nausea, hair loss, and, ironically, anemia, when I remembered I'd also face a more dangerous hurdle.

For one week or so of each three-week cycle, I'd endure the temporary destruction of my immune system. On those days, the microbes that we all carry, in our mouth, in our gut, and on our skin, (germs harmless to someone with a normal immune system), could precipitate a raging infection that could overwhelm and kill me in hours. The possibility of such an infection would tie me down geographically, because it meant I would have to remain within an hour of an emergency room at all times. And if I even thought I was running a fever, I'd have to report to the emergency room immediately for several days of intravenous antibiotics.

. . . .

AND THEN IT OCCURRED TO ME: THERE WAS ANOTHER CHOICE, A VERY OBVIOUS ONE.

. . . .

As a reward for my trouble, a few months of chemotherapy treatment would rid me of the night sweats, the fevers, and the daily flu. Maybe I'd be symptom-free for several more years. But eventually, chronic lymphocytic leukemia would come back for me. That gloomy fact kept hijacking my attention. I kept asking myself one question: Why was there no cure?

In fact the doctors had already answered that question for me. Their explanation went like this: chemotherapy would kill almost all of the leukemic cells in my body. But a few leukemic cells would be resistant to the drugs. Those resistant cells would survive the treatment, and would then gradually repopulate my marrow and blood with new—and resistant—leukemic cells. That was bad news. It meant that at some point in the future, not only would I become ill again, but my leukemia would have become "drug resistant."

While the real possibility of developing drug resistant disease was hardly a scenario I could get excited about, I did not toss out the possibility of having chemotherapy. Because as much as I wanted to live, I also wanted a life *worth* living. And at that moment, the life I was leading was not one I wanted to continue. I was dragging around, sick as a dog, unable to work more than an hour or so each day, unable to really enjoy anything. And so chemotherapy, with all its warts, was still on the table.

For the next week Linda and I talked about the mechanics of treatment, and what it would involve in terms of work, childcare, and caring for my aging parents, and the myriad other details that need to be considered before a cancer treatment protocol commences. Going to Boston for treatment with Dr. Nadler would be too difficult. That left Dr. Ambinder in Baltimore, or Dr. Kressel in Washington, D.C.

I decided to go with Dr. Kressel. He was a fine physician, skilled in his field, and I knew I could rely on him to give me an opinion that was both kind and scientific. However, I wasn't crazy about accepting his opinion, because it seemed amazingly gloomy. But I had no other choice.

And then it occurred to me: there was another choice, a very obvious one. This other choice would require the services of another type of healer. One who refused to buy into the pessimism of the medical establishment. One who didn't give a damn what others thought about pursuing the impossible. A healer willing to do research and look carefully at me, and at all possibilities for treating my chronic lymphocytic leukemia.

I didn't need to go far to find this healer. I had already met him. It was me.

I would have to learn how to treat myself. ❦

36

I HAD KEPT IN TOUCH with Irv Rosenberg throughout my setback. When he heard of my struggles, he reviewed my supplement protocol and recommended three additional nutraceuticals he thought I ought to try. The first was conjugated linoleic acid (CLA), a fatty acid found in high amounts in the fat of grass-fed cows. Animal studies suggested that CLA might be useful in cancer therapy, although trials in humans had not been done at the time. Still, Rosenberg thought supplemental CLA might be useful for me, because my near-vegetarian diet did not provide fat from beef or dairy.

The second additional nutraceutical Rosenberg recommended was a whey protein with lactoferrin, immunoglobulins, and other peptides. Rosenberg's third recommendation was that I take the botanical artemisinin. Long used as an antimalarial, artemisinin also exhibits anticancer activity. At the time of writing this book, artemisinin is the subject of brisk research.

I did my own reading on Rosenberg's three recommendations. The rationale sounded reasonable to me, and as there seemed to be little risk of serious side effects, I added the new supplements to my daily routine.

Meanwhile, my oncologists were pressing me to start treatment. *Real* treatment, as they called it. That term made me feel—perhaps unfairly—that they did not consider my home-cobbled program to be worth much consideration.

That was where our opinions differed. Some readers might wonder at this point whether I was seeing my situation clearly. I don't believe I was in denial about my condition; I understood how ill I was. But I also knew that I was in no immediate danger of going into a coma or dying, and that the conventional treatment promised little. Beyond that, I was stymied. So I did what my gut told me was wise: I stalled.

I told Dr. Kressel that I needed more time to think about treatment, that I was going to tough out my symptoms for a while, make some changes to my nutraceutical protocol, and see how that affected my blood.

Then I took a leap. Although it seems like a small leap in hindsight, it was a big leap at that moment! For me, and probably for a lot of other cancer patients as well, it would still be an almost unimaginable step. What did I do? I proposed a little research partnership between me and Dr. Kressel.

I proposed that together, Dr. Kressel and I monitor the anemia. I would revisit and reinforce my home-cobbled program, and would show up twice a week at his office for blood work. That way we'd have numbers—real data. We'd know for certain whether I was getting better or worse.

Dr. Kressel was game. The experiment was on! 🐝

37

THINGS WERE GOING WELL AT WORK. My very capable brother Jeff, and my publisher, Lee Mergner, had taken over the day-to-day running of *JazzTimes*. They and the other managers brought me only the most pressing problems, the ones only I could handle. Sick as I was, I managed to unfold a laptop and pound out an hour to two of work every day from bed.

Our advertising sales had rebounded nicely from the post-9/11 dip, and we had a new travel division that was growing nicely. The timing of this business upswing was fortunate, as it meant I could concentrate much of my daily effort on my health.

With Rosenberg's revised protocol in place, and having decided to delay chemotherapy, I thought long and hard about other beneficial lifestyle changes I could make.

Meanwhile the night sweats continued. So did the low-grade fevers, headaches, and a bone-wilting fatigue that took any exercise out of the equation—or so my physicians thought. Severe anemia puts a strain on the heart, even at rest, and exertion could be fatal. Although my anemia was only moderate, I really did feel more than wiped out.

However, I had an inkling that what was actually making the fatigue worse was lack of activity. Hard workouts were so much a part of my daily life that my body had become accustomed to them. Just a few days without exercise left me out of sorts. Going several weeks without exercise was depressing me.

The illness itself was debilitating, but to me, the inactivity seemed even more incapacitating. While this situation might seem like a contradiction, it was some years later before I learned of scientific evidence that explained what I was feeling. Research has shown that a single bout of resistance exercise (such as weightlifting) increases blood levels of a protein that neuroscientists have dubbed "brain-derived neurotrophic factor" (BDNF).[9] As the name suggests, BDNF promotes the growth of neurons and connections within the brain. BDNF's activity may partly explain why exercise is as potent an antidepressant as are pharmaceuticals.[10]

9 Yarrow JF, White LJ, McCoy SC, Borst SE.Training augments resistance exercise induced elevation of circulating brain derived neurotrophic factor (BDNF). Neurosci Lett. 2010 Jul 26;479(2):161-5.
10 Blumenthal JA, Babyak MA, Doraiswamy PM, Watkins L, Hoffman BM, Barbour KA et al. Exercise and pharmacotherapy in the treatment of major depressive disorder. Psychosom Med. 2007 Sep-Oct;69(7):587-96

Even though I hadn't heard of any such thing at the time, my body was giving me the message that I needed some vigorous exercise. Somehow, deep inside, I knew what I had to do.

I scraped myself out of bed, took a shower, dressed in some comfortable clothes, and announced to Linda that I was headed out for a walk. She wondered at first if I was kidding, but I grabbed Jazz's leash and the keys to the Goat.

· ·

LIFE WAS GOOD AGAIN, AND SO PRECIOUS. SPENDING TIME IN THE GRANDEUR OF NATURE MADE MY PROBLEMS SEEM MANAGEABLE.

· ·

The top was down, and I left it that way, even though it was summer and hot, and I was feverish and anemic and I should have stayed in air conditioning; even though CLL put me at higher risk for melanoma and I should have stayed out of direct sunlight. I needed that convertible ride. I needed it to feel alive again, to take back some morsel of control. Like the control I had regained at Sibley Memorial Hospital, when I took a little trip outside of the campus with my IV pole! Besides, Jazz loved to ride with the top down, and anticipating this, he had hopped into his usual shotgun post.

A moment later we were speeding toward Sligo Creek Park, Jazz's nose pointed into the wind. It had been much too long since either of us had taken a walk on our favorite patch of earth. I've mentioned Sligo Creek Park before, and how special it is to me. The paved trail runs north to south through two counties, with a 7 mile stretch in Montgomery County, where we live. This tree-shaded, creekside path is popular with walkers, joggers, and bikers; their company and my cell phone made me feel safe. This was no ordinary leisurely walk I was looking forward to. I was planning to go all out!

By the time I pulled into a parking spot at the park, Jazz was quivering so hard with excitement, I had trouble attaching the leash to his collar.

Then we were off, strolling under a canopy of trees, filtered light illuminating the trail. Fifteen minutes into our walk I was exhausted, and we turned back. At most we had covered only a mile, probably much less. But it was more than I had walked for weeks. We headed back home, where I plopped into bed for a nap.

I followed the same pattern of daily brisk walks for the next couple of weeks.

Life was good again, and so precious. Spending time in the grandeur of nature made my problems seem manageable.

Jazz was my friend in this endeavor. His enthusiasm made my walks longer, then faster. By the time we were covering more than a couple of miles in 45 minutes, my brain was firing on all cylinders. I was getting fresh air. My metabolism was speeding up. Sure, the walks were hard, but I didn't drop dead of a heart attack. The anemia, elevated temperature, fatigue, and night sweats continued, but despite this, I was physically active again. The exercise was helping me, physically and emotionally.

I timed my new exercise program to coincide with the blood tests Dr. Kressel and I had agreed on. I would walk into his office sweating, and banter jovially with the nurses, who could not believe I was out exercising in the intensely humid D.C. summer. Despite the wearisome symptoms I was enduring most of the time, during those moments in Dr. Kressel's office, I probably looked perfectly healthy. Unfortunately, the blood tests did not look so well. ♥

38

SEVERAL WEEKS INTO my revised nutraceutical and exercise program, my blood counts were what doctors call "stable." Translated, that means there was no change. If viewed positively, it meant that although my counts were still a mess, at least they weren't any worse. Indeed, I chose to view this situation as positive. And my response was to up the ante. If my exercise program wasn't working, I'd work harder. I would also add swimming to my exercise routine.

My first time in the water, I did about eight slow lengths in a 50-meter outdoor pool. The sun on my skin, and my arms cutting through the water felt amazing. But I was sucking air in so hard that when I finished, I had to chill in a poolside chair for an hour. Once I felt recovered from the exertion, I went home and picked up Jazz. He and I then headed to Sligo Creek Park for a nice outdoor walk. This was the first time in weeks that I had done back-to-back workouts in the same day. And I did them with my symptoms still raging.

Over the next weeks, as often as I could, I swam. I stretched too, one muscle group at a time, and I could feel the strength and spring return to my step. And the walks with Jazz were just glorious. The fresh oxygen, vivid green of the leaves, the sounds and view of the flowing creek, people out and about doing their thing, playing with their kids—wow! It sure as hell beat lying around in bed feeling sorry for myself. Even though I still felt so lousy, I was living!

To me, exercise was a healing form of meditation. Although the walks and swims were short, at least for the first month or so, they still happened every day. I began to view this lower impact exercise as "relaxational exercise."

While walking or swimming, my mind quieted. My thoughts melted away. I was simply being, with awareness and gratitude. When a thought entered my mind, I let it flow out again, and I did not cling to it. Instead, I visualized oxygen, sun, and my metabolism decimating the leukemia cells traveling through my bloodstream.

The warmth of the summer sunlight made exercise all the more powerful. In winter, my outdoor activity would have been limited, and I am not convinced I would have stayed the course I had set out for myself. I might have gone with the conventional chemotherapy.

Then there was my family. Linda fed me the most wonderful food and helped me keep my spirits up. Little Jared was a joy—sweet, cuddly, and a toddler too young to know what was going on. But Miles was seven. He could not really understand why I was too sick to play catch or soccer with him, yet he saw me going for walks and swims. How confusing that must have been for him. How could he possibly understand that exercise was a key part of my therapy, and that I had to make it a priority? I felt for Miles. But I knew that the choices I made, I made for him. I wanted to live. For him.

I stayed the course. I proceeded with my self-directed program of activity, declining conventional treatment. I went to Dr. Kressel regularly for blood tests, as he and I had agreed. As I mentioned above, for the first weeks, the results showed no improvement. Although no worse, I was just as anemic as ever.

And then, during the third week, Dr. Kressel and I got a surprise. ♥

39

THERE WAS A MEASURABLE IMPROVEMENT in my counts! That initial result was good, Dr. Kressel explained, but caution was needed. To prove this result was a trend, we'd need three consecutive tests showing improvement. I was to return a week later, for the second of the three tests.

I left Dr. Kressel's office cautiously optimistic. Well, no, that's not quite true. Hell no, I was ecstatic! My self-directed program was—in my mind at least—working! I began to push even harder. I sped up my walks, and I lengthened my swims. I adhered to my entire regimen like my life depended on it, and perhaps it did.

The following week I was back at Dr. Kressel's for another blood test. When I heard the result, I joyfully blurted out "another improvement!" Dr. Kressel, ever the rigorous physician, cautioned that this was indeed a slight improvement.

Caution was not what I was about at that moment. I allowed myself to be wildly, irresponsibly, encouraged. I still felt ill, but I was making progress! From the doctor's office, I went home, scooped up Jazz and headed directly to Sligo Creek Park. We had a nice—and very long—walk.

The fourth and fifth week's blood tests confirmed we had a trend. The anemia was definitely improving. Although my red cell levels were not back to normal, they were definitely on their way. And the improvement was happening without prednisone or chemotherapy.

I continued twice weekly blood tests. I was exercising more and more. I was feeling somewhat better. The blood tests continued to improve.

But something was still very wrong. I was still having fevers. I was still having night sweats. The leukemia was still active. 🐾

40

AND THEN, SEVERAL MONTHS AFTER the fevers began, they went away. My night sweats vanished. My blood counts completely normalized.

I had faced down the leukemia. It had backed off. I was out of immediate danger!

Dr. Kressel was pleased by the complete turnaround in my condition, although he could not explain what had happened. He recommended we take a closer look at my blood using a technique called flow cytometry. This investigation would tell us if leukemic cells were still lurking among the normal blood cells.

Within a few days I got the results.

They nearly floored me.

There were no leukemic cells in my blood.

None. 🖤

41

AS ANXIOUS AS I WAS to tell Dr. Nadler the news, my first calls were to Linda, my parents, and Irv Rosenberg. Although Rosenberg is not easily excited, he was happy to hear the results. I thanked him for all his support. In my mind, his revisions to my protocol had played a large role in my recovery.

It seemed to me that there was a powerful, synergistic effect between the nutraceutical compounds, my diet, physical activity, and my improving health. Perhaps consistent daily exercise contributed to an increased metabolic rate, and maybe my stress hormones were kept in check through all of these things. Ultimately, my body's innate healing capacity was activated. I can't know exactly how this came about. I can only speculate that my lifestyle played a big part. Whatever the molecular details, I knew I had accomplished something important. This achievement was beyond empowering.

When I got Dr. Nadler on the phone I began to rattle off the particulars about my somewhat amateur—but wildly successful—supplement, exercise and diet program, my "n-of-1" experiment.

Dr. Nadler's excitement was palpable. He had previously seen with his own eyes how sick I was. He was dumbfounded at hearing of my recovery, and without treatment—or to be more precise, without "standard" treatment, meaning chemotherapy. He asked to see me in clinic as soon as possible, so he could run some tests to confirm my recovery. And, to my surprise and joy, he wanted to learn more about my program. ❦

42

A TRIP TO BOSTON WOULD HAVE TO WAIT. Though my condition had improved, I was in no shape to travel. Although the headaches, fevers, and night sweats were gone, I was still exhausted. I was weak and thin once again, which brought back memories of the time after the splenectomy in 1992. So I set out to regain vitality in my usual way. ❦

43

ON MY FIRST DAY BACK AT THE GYM I was met with exclamations of "Wow, you've lost a lot of weight!" and "Are you okay?" Truth be told, I was not OK.

A 20-minute workout left me sore for days. But I knew the drill, and a gradual increase in the duration and frequency of my workouts soon had me putting on muscle.

About this same time, I returned to work full time. Although I had kept working part-time throughout my illness, I had a lot of catching up to do, and I had to muster some discipline to balance work and health. I still got to the gym daily, and, with Linda, kept up with family life. Miles, seven, and Jared, almost two, were our great joys. And of course there was Jazz.

But then Jazz stopped going with me on walks. He stared bleakly at his heaping food bowl, refusing to eat. I took him to the vet, and after the veterinarian ran some tests, he walked in with bad news.

Jazz had kidney cancer. 🐾

44

JAZZ WAS OUR "FIRST BORN." Linda and I had gotten him a few weeks before our wedding. I had always envisioned playing Frisbee with a big-boned lab. But Linda won the argument about the size of dog we should get, and so a small dog it was. In responding to the advertisement, we found ourselves in a seedy Baltimore neighborhood, peering at a squirming litter of miniature schnauzer puppies. Linda chose a particularly wiggly pup, one with brown eyes as liquid and deep as love. We named him *Jazz*. Within a few weeks I was hopelessly in love with that dog.

Now Jazz was sick, and we decided to have the veterinarian remove his cancerous kidney. We spent the next days tending night and day to our beloved little Jazz, providing round the clock care that included pain meds, subcutaneous fluid injections, the works.

He held on for a week. Then our beautiful little Jazz, our firstborn, left us. Linda and I mourned. 🌱

45

ALMOST THREE YEARS TICKED BY, and my blood tests remained normal, so I finally made an appointment to see Dr. Nadler in Boston. It was late spring, 2006, and I had worked out extra hard a couple of weeks before, just to make sure I looked my best. I could not wait to show off my regained health, and to get Dr. Nadler's take on my *n*-of-1 health program.

After a full day of blood tests and scans, I sat fidgeting with excitement in Dr. Nadler's waiting room. I could hardly wait to see his reaction when he saw me. At my last appointment, I had been so ill. I was feverish, weak, and closer to death than I had ever been. Now, not only was I was pumped with new muscle, I was energetic, and confident to the point of cockiness.

The first thing Dr. Nadler said when he walked into the lobby to summon me was how good I looked! In the exam room he pressed his stethoscope to my chest to listen to my heart and lungs: normal. He palpated my neck and underarms for swollen lymph nodes: normal. He went to his computer to view the results of the morning's blood tests and scans. He frowned at the screen, looked at me, and then once again scrutinized the screen, and shook his head.

Dr. Nadler pulled up the report from my previous visit in summer of 2003, when I'd been so ill. He stared at it, and shook his head again. He told me that in his 30 years as a doctor, he had never encountered a patient with CLL who had done so well. My recovery was—it seemed—rather remarkable.

"Am I a freak of nature?" I asked, only half joking. Dr. Nadler shook his head in disbelief.

"You're a *force* of nature!" he replied.

There was no evidence of leukemia on *any* of the tests, he told me. "You willed it away." Dr. Nadler told me that patients who are involved in their care generally do much better than those who have a more passive approach to their illness. How, I recall him wondering aloud, had I done it? ❦

46

IT SEEMED TO ME that Dr. Nadler thought that my remission must have been attributable to one thing in my protocol. One supplement or one botanical had to be responsible for the stunning turnaround in my health. Dr. Nadler wanted to know exactly which one it was.

I was more than happy to spend the next 45 minutes explaining to Dr. Nadler all the things I had done: my incredibly healthy diet, the meditative walks, the long swims, the weight workouts, and the nutraceuticals program.

The nutraceuticals caught Dr. Nadler's attention. He made me go over them several times, while he took notes and asked questions about formulations, dosages, and schedules.

In contrast to Dr. Nadler's formal medical training, I didn't know a molecule from a manatee! But what I lacked in scientific and medical education, I made up for in spades in the swagger department. I told Dr. Nadler, point blank, that I thought that looking for one active agent responsible for my recovery was the wrong approach. In my opinion, the secret formula was the *combination* of diet, exercise, mind-body work, and nutraceuticals.

Whatever Dr. Nadler, the Harvard professor, thought about this challenge from a guy whose biology education had taken place at the gym, he was genial about it. ❧

47

THE BLOOD TEST RESULTS should have been good news. And indeed they were, but all was not entirely settled. Though I was ecstatic that the blood tests showed no leukemic cells, and the scans no swollen lymph nodes, I knew that leukemia is ultimately a disease of the bone marrow. The leukemic cells originate in the marrow, and from the marrow they migrate into the blood. The absence of leukemic cells in my blood was a very good sign. But if there were still leukemic cells in my marrow, the disease would come back. Only if the marrow itself was clear of leukemic cells could I be considered to be in "complete" or "pathologic remission."

Deep down in my heart, clear marrow was what I wanted. I wanted to be free of leukemia once and for all. If I wanted to know if I was indeed "cured," I would have to take the only test that would tell me what was happening deep in my bones—another bone marrow biopsy.

Something inside me gathered the chutzpah to ask Dr. Nadler to do a bone marrow biopsy.

He refused. He explained that the results of a bone marrow biopsy wouldn't change any treatment decisions, because even if the biopsy showed leukemic cells lingering in my marrow, it was clear that I did not need treatment at the moment.

Dr. Nadler was correct, of course. The results of the bone marrow biopsy would not change the conventional approach to my treatment. Conventional medicine treated CLL patients only to control symptoms, and since I was no longer having symptoms, I did not require treatment. Why put a patient through a painful test, with risks of bleeding, infection, and perhaps also of the needle breaking off in the bone, if the results wouldn't change the treatment approach?

But to me, the knowledge resulting from a new bone marrow biopsy mattered. The results mattered to me a lot.

So I pressed Dr. Nadler to do the biopsy. Other than the usual risks of bleeding, infection and so on—risks I was fully prepared to take—what harm could come of it?

Dr. Nadler is a wise man. He explained that there was indeed a chance of harm, a very big chance. Psychological and emotional harm could come to me if the biopsy revealed persistent leukemia. He urged me instead to relax, to enjoy the elation of success. Why ruin the moment just to satisfy my curiosity?

That argument gave me pause. I had not seriously considered the psychological impact of unpleasant test results in the past, nor could I recall discussing this topic with any other physicians.

Of course, I was also aware of the subtext. Dr. Nadler may have felt certain that my marrow harbored leukemic cells, although I never asked him. That belief would have been justified by existing medical knowledge of the disease. CLL didn't simply go away. No one had been cured of this disease, either with conventional treatment, or with any other approach.

At that point I was 12 years into my illness, and almost as many years into my experiment. I was heady with confidence, because I had won a battle with CLL, and without using conventional treatment.

I had come this far only by keeping my eyes wide open. Closing them now hardly seemed wise. Keeping my eyes open meant a bone marrow biopsy. I wanted to look into my own marrow, to face my leukemia opponent head on. I wanted to know how deep my remission was.

Even as Dr. Nadler was making his exit, I began to scheme. How could I get a bone marrow biopsy done if he was not prepared to do it? And if I did have the procedure, and leukemic cells indeed lurked in my marrow, was Dr. Nadler right about the psychological and emotional impact of the results? Would knowledge wound me?

48

LIKE MOST PEOPLE, I prefer to keep up a front of bravado. However, I knew that emotional trauma was all too real, and that Dr. Nadler's warning required my attention.

Once home in Maryland, I rehearsed in my mind how it would feel to get the results of the bone marrow biopsy. It didn't take much introspection to come to a conclusion. After the recent elation of the perfect blood tests, learning that leukemia still lurked in my bone marrow—and in my future—would be tough.

But I had a burning curiosity that I just couldn't shake. What if the unheard of had indeed happened? What if my health program had actually contributed to clearing the leukemia out of my marrow? Although it would be impossible to prove cause and effect, I felt it was crucial to know exactly what was going on in my bone marrow. I knew that the scenario of leukemia-free marrow was very unlikely. I had never heard of that happening before. Perhaps even more importantly, my world-class oncologists had never heard of that happening. But there is a first time for everything, right? Isn't all human progress driven by curiosity, by a willingness to explore at the edge of what is thought possible, and by the courage to risk failure?

I was now a citizen scientist. Amateur yes, I knew. Hardly a world-renowned figure in my adopted field of CLL. But, I was determined not to be amateurish. I was absolutely serious about my research. I was conducting a study with an *n* of 1, the most precious single sample, myself. I had vowed to learn as much as I could about my body and my health. And in my opinion, a bone marrow biopsy, although not medically indicated, was scientifically indicated.

While one part of me was determined to demand a bone marrow biopsy, a second part of me worried about the emotional consequences, and a third part of me looked on with amazement. I, Glenn Sabin, was disagreeing with Dr. Nadler, one of the world's most respected oncologists in the field of CLL. Who was I to think that I knew better than he about anything related to this awful disease?

On the other hand, I was a bona fide expert, at least when it came to my own bloodstream. Had my own leukemia backed down? If so, did this have something to do with diet, exercise, stress reduction, psychosocial support, and targeted nutraceuticals? I had data that suggested just that. And that data made me hungry for more. I would insist upon having a bone marrow biopsy. I would find out if my marrow contained leukemic cells.

In the end it was Dr. Kressel who agreed to do the procedure. I went to his office early on a weekday morning, lay face down on the exam table, and winced as he stuck a six-inch needle into the back of my hipbone. I was satisfied with my decision. I knew in my gut it was the right one.

The phone call came a week later. The results were in. 🌱

49

LEUKEMIC CELLS WERE STILL THERE, lurking deep in my marrow. The news was a brutal kick to the stomach of Glenn-the-patient.

So Glenn-the-investigator stepped in. I would get a second opinion. I immediately made arrangements to have the marrow specimen sent to the Dana-Farber Cancer Institute for examination.

The results were the same: leukemia.

When Dr. Nadler phoned to ask how I was doing with the news, I tried to hide my devastation. Managing an even tone, I told him that of course I was disappointed.

Dr. Nadler told me I shouldn't be. The most advanced chemotherapy could not have produced a better response. Even with the most advanced chemotherapy, I would almost certainly still have had leukemic cells in my bone marrow. Dr. Nadler explained that the course of my CLL thus far had been so extraordinary, considering that I was feeling better, and all without conventional therapy.

Dr. Nadler explained that he had made arrangements for me to meet with someone very special. That someone was another Harvard professor, and director of perhaps the most unusual department within the cancer center. 🌱

50

DR. DAVID ROSENTHAL IS a fit, silver-haired man with clear blue eyes, elegant manners, and several decades of experience treating blood disorders. What was most unusual about his career, however, was the strange turn it had taken. In 2000, Dr. Rosenthal had inaugurated the first integrative medicine clinic[11] at the Dana-Farber Cancer Institute, and in 2003, he and two other academics had founded the Society for Integrative Oncology.

In academic centers, integrative therapies are promoted as providing symptom relief only. Any implication that diet, exercise, stress reduction, or other "alternative" therapies might in themselves enhance survival is largely avoided.

Dr. Rosenthal had set up a modest integrative medicine clinic right in the center of Harvard's Dana-Farber Cancer Institute, complete with massage therapists, nutritionists, and Chinese medicine practitioners. Two days a week he saw patients there, and the rest of the week he continued his mainstream medical duties in the hematology department.

Dr. Rosenthal leaned forward as I told him my story. When I finished, he looked at me thoughtfully. Then he told me about the one case of "spontaneous remission" of CLL he had seen. It had happened some 25 years before. The gentleman had a high fever from CLL. He was preparing for an autologous bone marrow transplant but decided to delay the procedure in order to bank his sperm. During the two weeks it took to get that done, the fever dissipated and he went into clinical remission. What eventually became of the gentleman, Rosenberg did not know.

My interactions with Dr. Rosenberg and Dr. Nadler, and their interest in my endeavors, gave me a new kind of confidence.

I began to see that my story might benefit other cancer patients, and I felt a large responsibility. I began to pour everything into getting my story out: my money, my time, and most of all, my dreams. ♠

---

11 Zakim Center marks progress and promise of integrative therapies for cancer patients. Available at: http://www.dana-farber.org/Newsroom/Publications/Zakim-Center-marks-progress-and-promise-of-integra-tive-therapies-for-cancer-patients.aspx (http://bit.ly/2cFD61q)

51

OVER THE NEXT FEW YEARS, I began to tell my story. This was a casual endeavor, and some CLL patients sought me out for further information. I simply shared the basic principles of health that I followed: drinking lots of water, exercising regularly, practicing meditation or mindfulness in ways that worked best for me, and eating a plant-strong, chemical-free, whole foods diet. This mixture was hardly rocket science. Most people had heard these things, and already knew that health habits were important. I saw my job at that time as being a living example of what might be possible if those theories were actually put into practice.

When someone pressed me for more specific information, I asked them to request their doctor's approval, and only when this was obtained, I asked them to do three things faithfully: drink plenty of clean water each day, take a 30-40 minute walk daily, and cut out all sugared beverages. If they actually stuck to this for three weeks, and noticed that they felt better, they could call back. Then we'd discuss diet, specifically lightening up on animal products, and emphasizing whole foods, vegetables, and fruits. I'd also suggest reading materials I'd found helpful.

I didn't know it then, but I was beginning a brand new career. Taking control of my health had shifted the center of my professional life, from the media business to promoting integrative medicine.

Meanwhile, the arrival of the internet had brought big changes to our media business. I worked hard to move *JazzTimes* into this new era, by acquiring a new magazine, producing award-winning journalism and graphic design, creating dynamic new websites, and growing the travel and custom publishing divisions. However, even these changes were not enough to prop up a business that heavily relied on print advertising. *JazzTimes* struggled, and after 25 years at the helm of the operation, I decided to put the business on the market.

I needed to support my young family, and so I started looking for a new path. I didn't have to look far. I brimmed with a new passion, and I wanted to help anyone who was struggling with cancer. I wanted physicians to be convinced that lifestyle mattered, so that they could encourage their patients to make changes with more confidence. I wanted to advance the field of integrative medicine. Specifically, I wanted to make it available to anyone, anywhere. I wanted to make integrative medicine the new standard of care.

That goal would prove almost as impossible to achieve as curing myself of leukemia at home. As usual, my ignorance of that fact was what allowed me to proceed. ❦

IN 2005, LINDA TORE A PAGE from a magazine and set it on the pile on my nightstand. I picked it up and read it before I went to bed. It was a small news article about the use of something called EGCG that was being studied at the Mayo Clinic in Rochester, Minnesota. Epigallocatechin-3-gallate, (EGCG), is an alkaloid abundant in green tea. Mounting scientific evidence demonstrates its promise in treating many chronic disorders, including some forms of cancer. The article Linda had found described a study showing EGCG to be effective at killing CLL cells in a test tube.

I knew that it was easy to kill cancer cells in a test tube. However, the real test of any potential cancer treatment was how it performs in human beings. Although the EGCG study was a limited test tube study, it was certainly interesting! The next morning, I emailed the lead investigator, Dr. Neil Kay, told him my story, and asked what else his team was working on in terms of EGCG and CLL. Soon I was on the phone with him.

As luck would have it, the Mayo Clinic was recruiting CLL patients for a phase I clinical trial of EGCG. Excited, I asked for more details. Dr. Kay told me that ECGC was non-toxic, and that the clinical study would probably use doses of up to 4 grams per day. He asked if I was interested in volunteering. I certainly was!

Dr. Kay was planning to recruit between 45 and 75 CLL patients. There were two preconditions for participation in the trail. First, a subject must never have received conventional treatment for the disease. No problem, I thought. Second, a subject had to commit to going to Minnesota once a month for six months. *That* was a problem. Trekking to Minnesota during winter was not on my bucket list!

There was a further problem from my perspective. A phase I clinical trial, I knew by then, was primarily designed to test a drug's toxicity. A first group of patients would get a small dose of the drug being tested, and if they did okay, the next group of patients would receive a higher dose, the next group yet a higher dose, and so on, with that scheme being repeated until the side effects became intolerable, or the maximum dose, in Dr. Kay's study, 4 grams per day of EGCG, had been administered.

Any response to treatment was a secondary goal. I could see a problem there in my case. My counts were perfect and I felt entirely well, so it would have been impossible for Dr. Kay to know if the EGCG was actually benefiting me. I considered adding EGCG to my regimen on my own. But in the end I decided against it. Taking something I might not need was not my style.

That was in 2005, and although I declined to enter the Mayo study, I decided to keep in touch with Dr. Kay and his work. Because what if someday I needed EGCG? ❦

53

BY 2009, I WAS SPENDING MOST OF MY FREE TIME attending medical conferences. At these events I spoke to many doctors who wanted to practice integrative medicine, but who couldn't manage to make ends meet doing that work. When I saw how hard these physicians struggled with the business side of their practices, I felt for them. Then something clicked. Business was something I knew inside out; I could help. Soon I was putting together my own business plan.

As I pondered possible names for my new endeavor, Dr. Nadler's "Force of Nature" comment came to mind. Nature was indeed my medicine, and what a force it was! The phrase would not only communicate the spirit of the business, it would energize me whenever the going got tough. But "Force of Nature" as a name was too long. And that's how FON Therapeutics, since renamed FON Consulting, was born.

That naming matter being settled, I laid out the path my new endeavor would take. I would serve cancer patients, and their physicians and other practitioners. Together we would advance the field of integrative medicine.

It was as if I'd come home. 🌱

54

IT WASN'T UNTIL 2010 that FON found its core clientele, and it wasn't patients. Instead, FON would focus on the physicians devoted to providing integrative medicine to their patients. Focusing on the business of integrative medicine, I turned my efforts toward helping doctors, clinics, and academic centers develop and market integrative medicine programs.

As for my personal story, I continued working with Irv Rosenberg, was faithful to my diet and exercise program, and enjoyed my young family. Despite a challenging schedule, my health held up. And about this time I began hearing a new name: Dr. Keith Block. ❦

55

TWO PHRASES, "The Block Center," and "exemplary model of cancer care," kept appearing in the same sentence. Keith Block, MD, was the man behind this phenomenon, and I needed to become acquainted with this leader in integrative oncology. So when I found out he would be lecturing at a conference I was planning to attend, I composed an email to him, telling him of my story, and asking to meet briefly. It was a long shot, and I was not really expecting a positive response.

In fact, I knew I'd be lucky to get any response at all. Doctors are always busy, and I knew it, even as I pressed the "send" button.

To my surprise, the return email came almost immediately. Dr. Block's response was "Yes." ❧

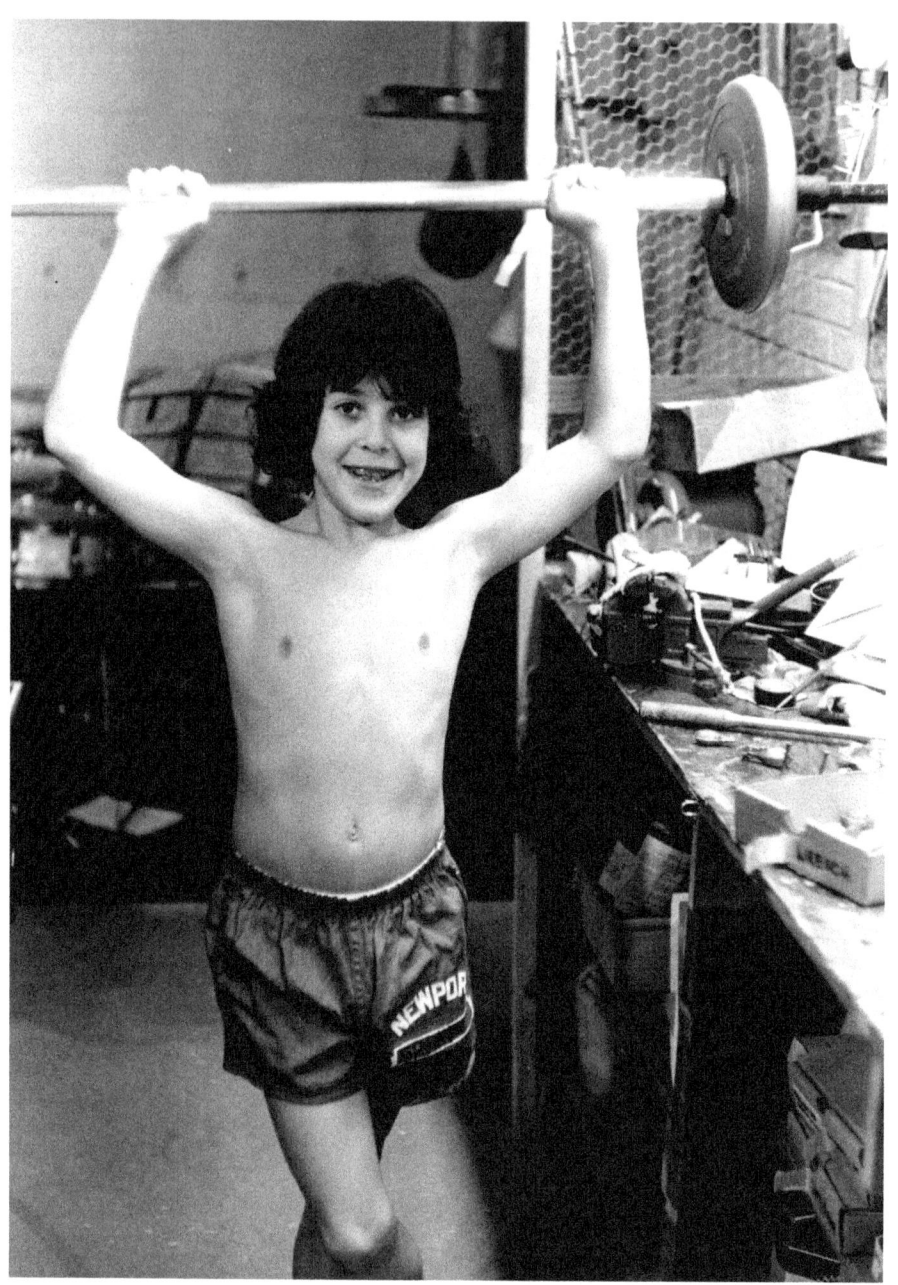

Glenn lifting weights at 12 years old, 1975

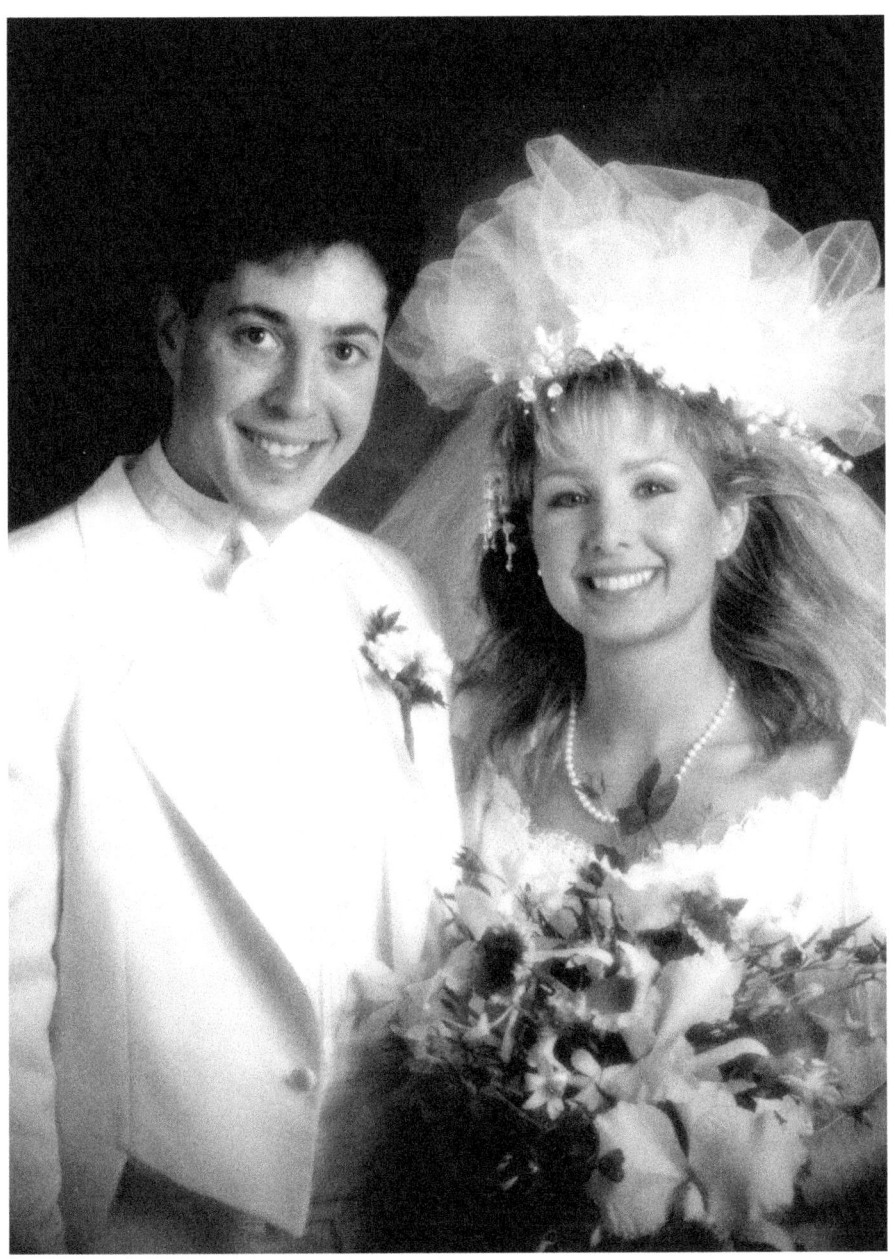

Our wedding day, 1989

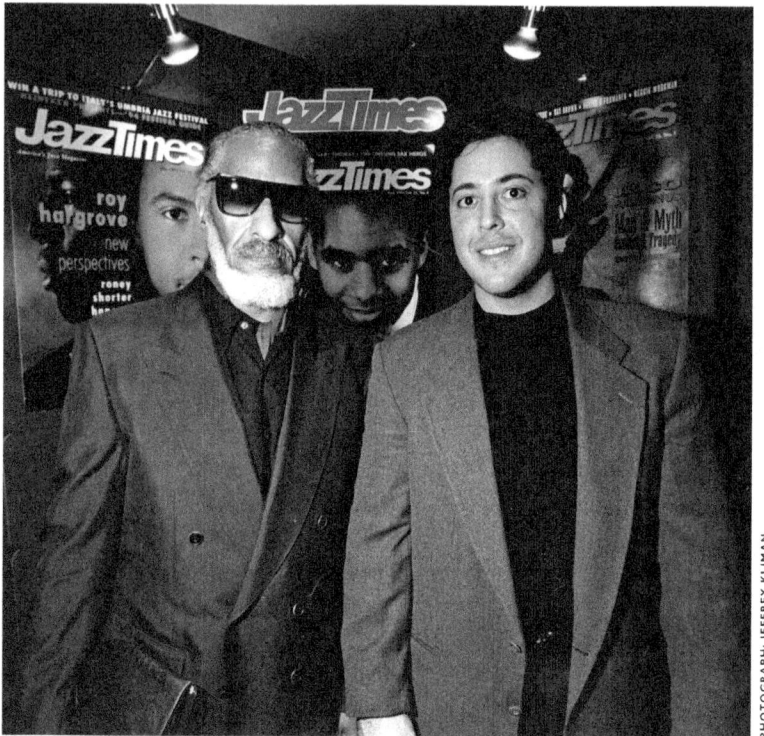

With jazz legend Sonny Rollins during *JazzTimes* Convention, New York City, 1994

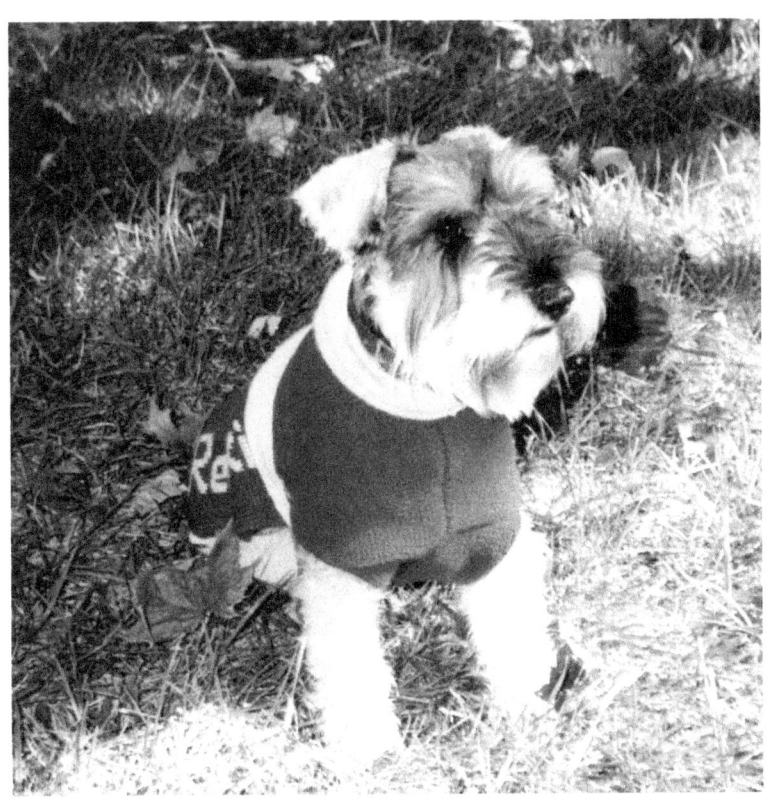

Jazz Sabin, 2003

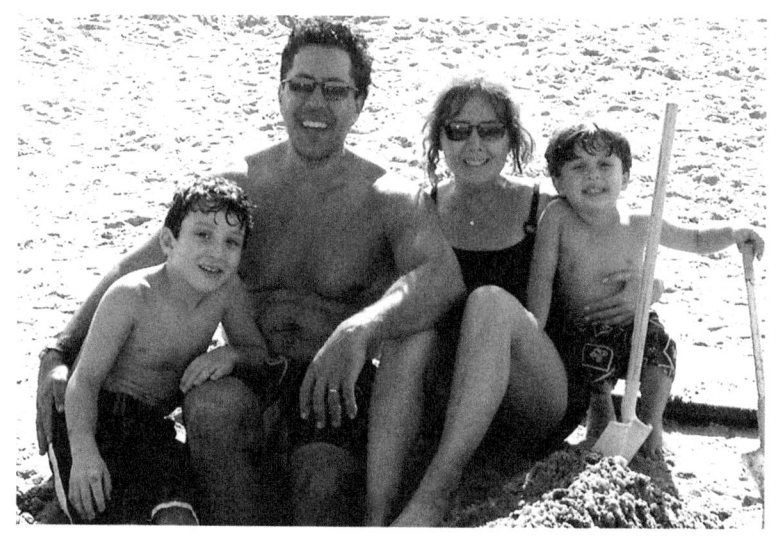

From Left: Miles, Glenn, Linda, and Jared Sabin, Rehoboth Beach, Delaware, 2005

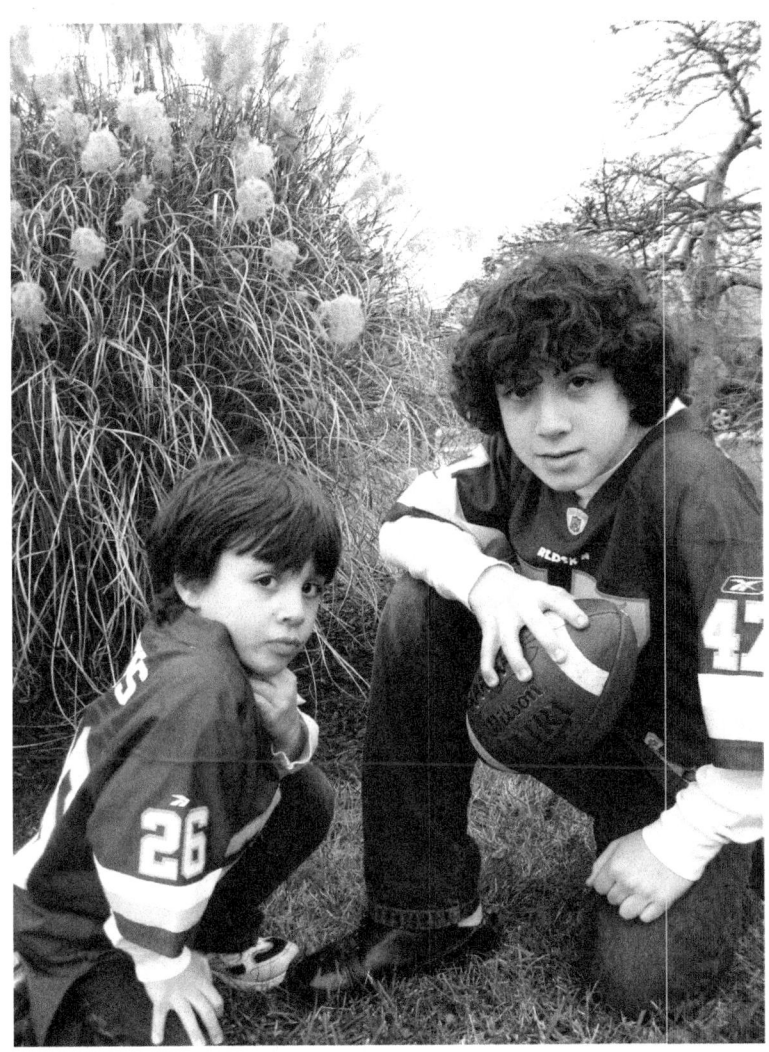

From left: Jared and Miles Sabin, 2008

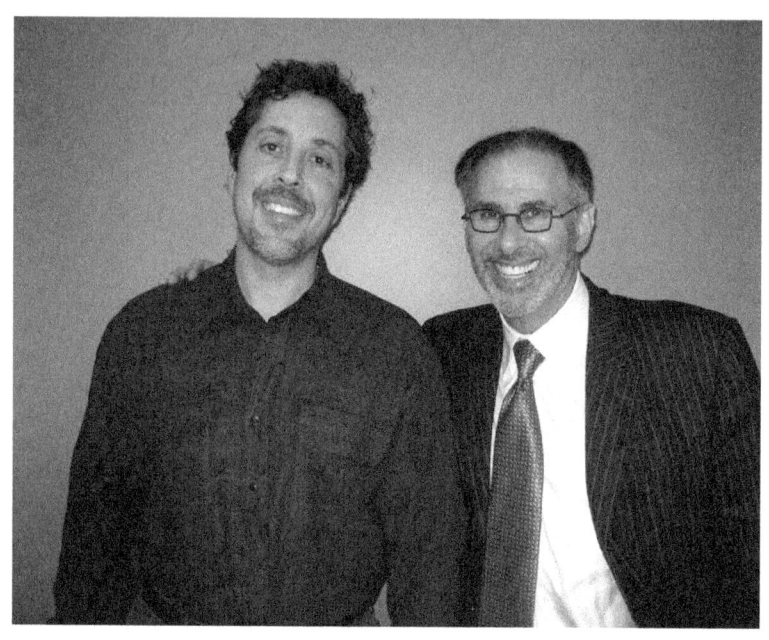

With Lee M. Nadler, MD, at Dana-Farber Cancer Institute, Boston, 2012

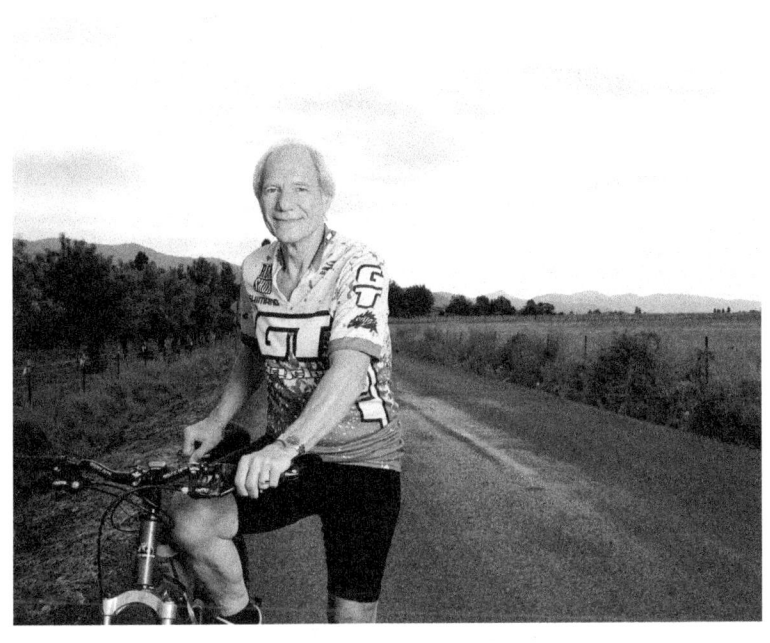

Ross Pelton, Ashland, Oregon, 2014

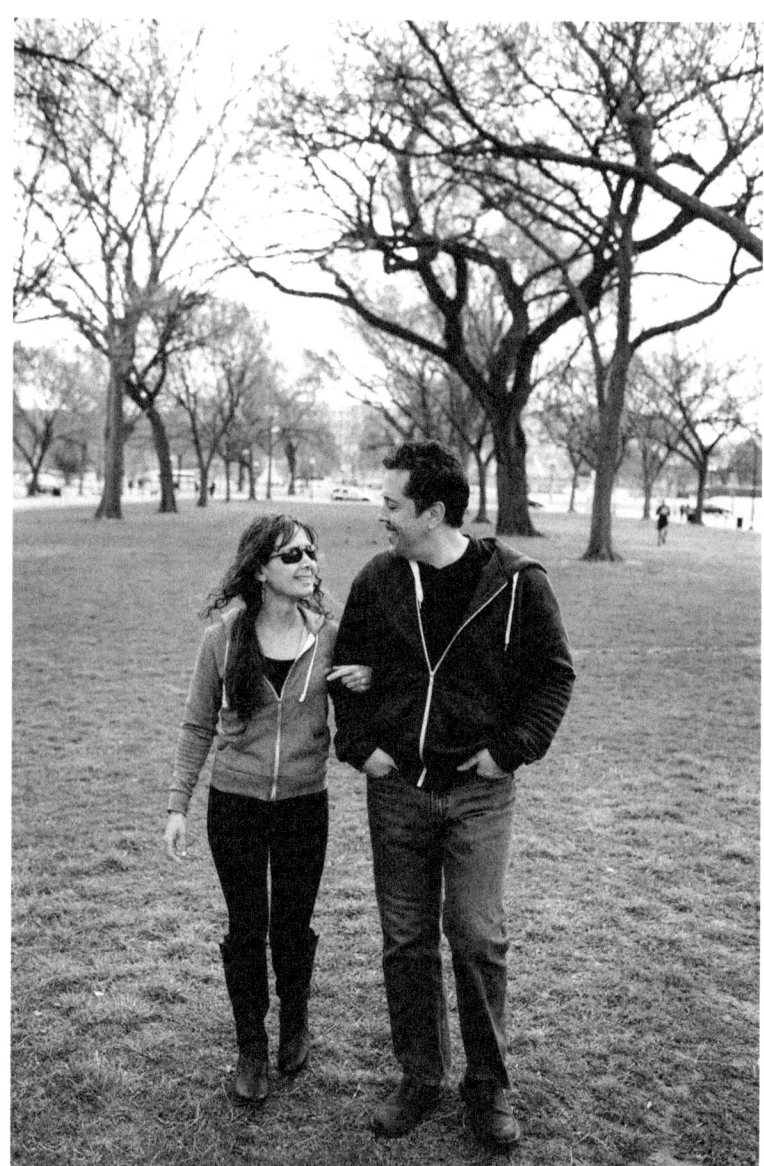

With Linda at the National Mall, Washington, D.C., 2015

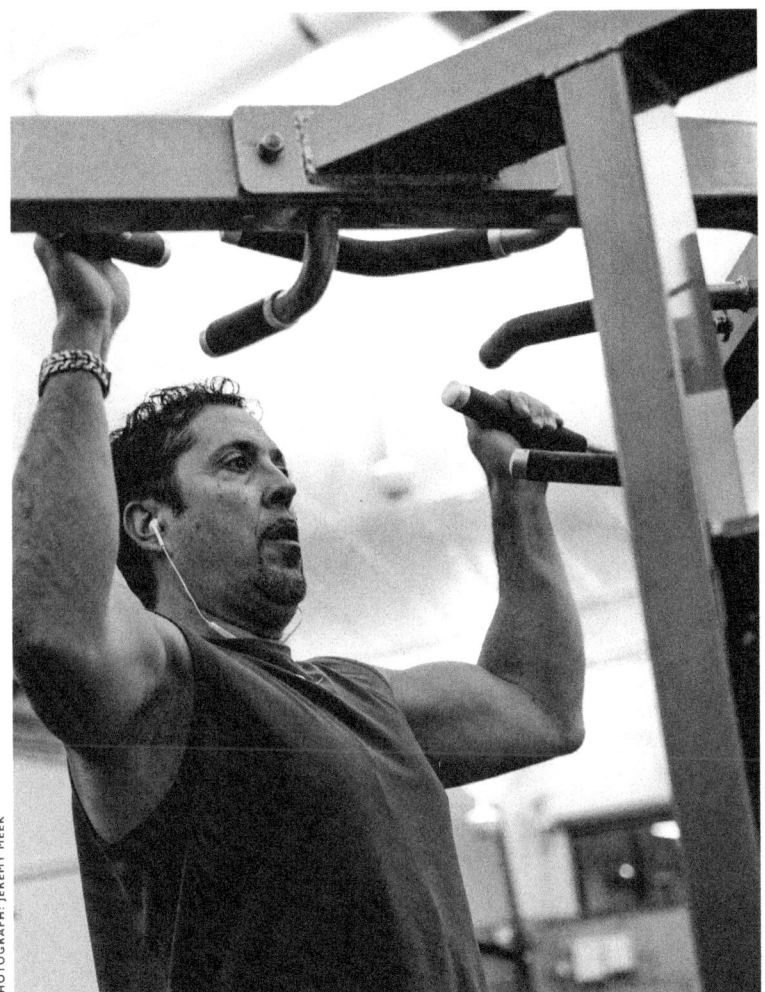

At The Aspen Hill Club, 2015

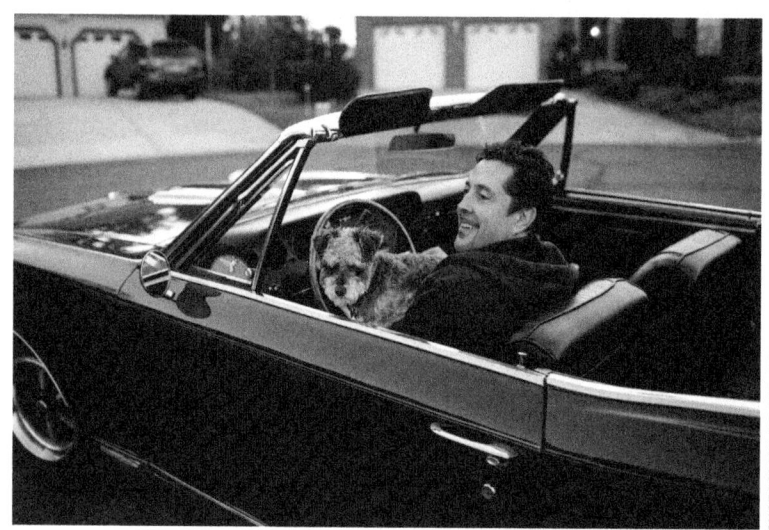

With new puppy Leo in my 1967 Pontiac GTO, 2015

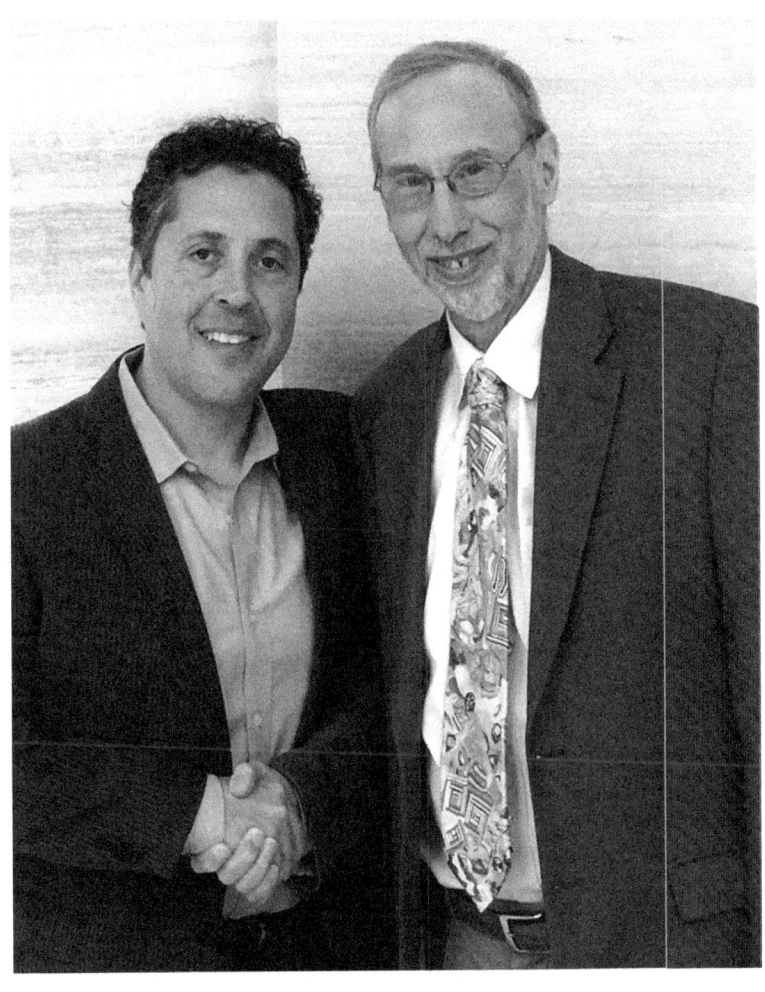

With Bruce R. Kressel, MD, at Johns Hopkins Sibley Memorial Hospital,
Washington, D.C., 2016

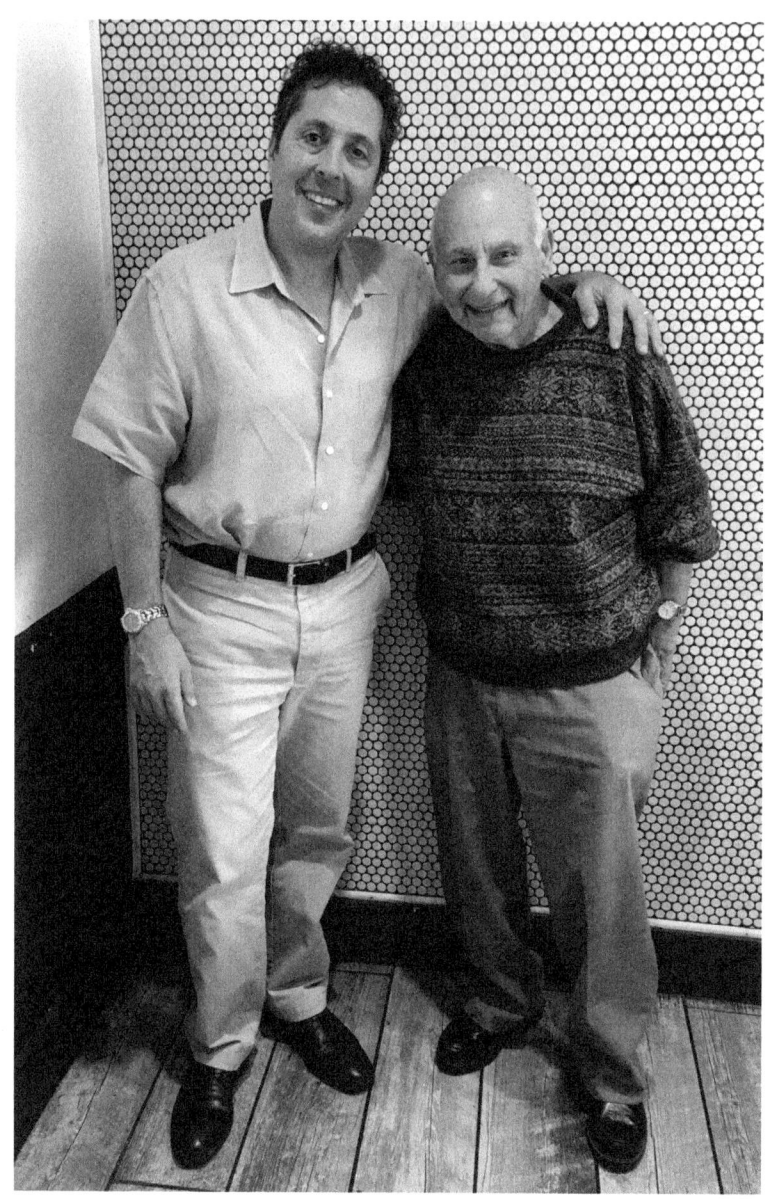

With Irwin "Irv" Rosenberg, 2016

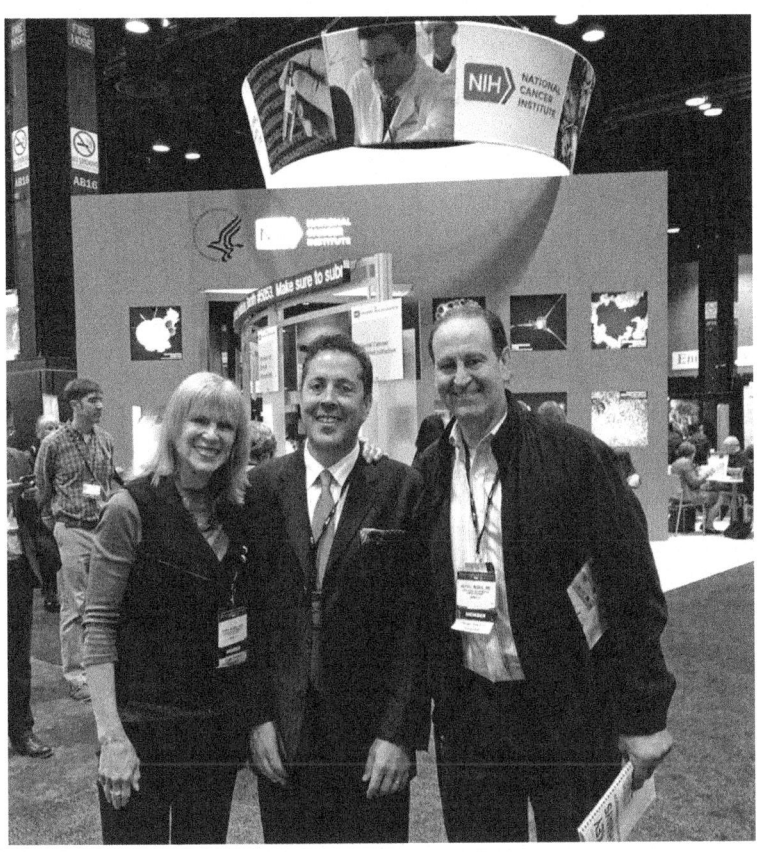

With Drs. Keith and Penny Block at the ASCO Annual Meeting, Chicago, 2016

• PART III •

N OF 1?

56

ATTENDING MEDICAL CONFERENCES would become part of my self-directed education, and the first I chose to attend was "Cancer Guides II," which was held in June 2009 at a large hotel in Washington, D.C. The conference was part of a series called "Cancer Guides" produced every few years by the Center for Mind-Body Medicine, based in Washington. I had heard about the conference from a colleague.

This conference was for medical professionals, not people like me. As I registered in the lobby outside the conference hall, I worried that I was in over my head. This lack of self-confidence was rare for me. It came about because I was really distracted. I was in the midst of selling the family business, a company I'd led for a quarter century. Negotiations were at a fevered pitch, and phone calls and emails were flying at a horrid pace. Getting through a lecture undisturbed was practically impossible. To say my attention was strained would be an understatement.

I prepared for the conference for months. I made a list of every researcher, clinician, or advocate whose lecture I wanted to hear, and emailed them, asking for a meeting. It sounds like a lot of work, and it was, but once I got going, the stars aligned. About a dozen people I wrote to responded, agreeing to meet with me.

Among those who replied was Dr. Harvey Fineberg, then president of the Institute of Medicine. He led me to Jacqueline Tschernia, a high-energy, passionate, and most effective cancer advocate. She in turn connected me with many more people who would help me in my quest. A snowball had begun. ❦

57

THE CONFERENCE was one of many produced by Dr. James Gordon. Dr. Gordon is a Harvard-educated psychiatrist, long at the forefront of education and advocacy for complementary and alternative, and now, integrative, medicine. He is well known as the founder and leader of D.C.'s Center for Mind-Body Medicine. Dr. Gordon has a curriculum vita that is long and impressive, including serving as a recent Chair of the White House Commission on Complementary and Alternative Medicine Policy.

Another prominent attendee at "Cancer Guides II" was David Servan-Schreiber, MD, PhD. Dr. Servan-Schreiber was the author of *Anticancer: A New Way of Life*. This book details the nutritional and lifestyle measures to which he attributed his 20-year survival, with what should have been a quickly fatal brain cancer.

Dr. Servan-Shreiber was a psychiatrist and neuroscientist at the University of Pittsburgh. He was also a driven man, one who lets nothing slow down his research schedules. As an illustration of this commitment, is the story of how Dr. Servan-Schreiber responded when a subject from the "normals" group didn't show up for a required brain scan. Instead of postponing the scan to track down the miscreant, Dr. Servan-Schreiber volunteered for a scan himself. However, much to everyone's horror, the scan showed that Dr. Servan-Schreiber's brain was not normal. It contained a large tumor.

To make a long story short, the tumor in Dr. Servan-Schreiber's brain was cancer. He underwent brain surgery and radiation therapy. He admits in the book that his first go-around with cancer didn't set off many alarm bells. After the surgery and radiation, Servan-Schreiber continued his unhealthy lifestyle, long hours, bad food, unnecessary stress, and lack of exercise.

A few years later, the tumor reappeared.

The relapse spurred Dr. Servan-Schreiber to investigate, and eventually adopt, extensive lifestyle interventions, including a plant-based diet, regular exercise, and restorative sleep.

What an encouraging confirmation of my experiences! I wrote to him to thank him for writing the book, and asked for a meeting.

And that was how Linda and I came to be eating lunch with Dr. Servan-Schreiber during the conference. He seemed eager to hear my thoughts on his work. I was even more eager to tell him! I told him that I thought his book was wonderful, but would have liked more emphasis on vigorous exercise, hydration, and well-placed nutraceuticals. I expressed my concern about the high inflammation and oxidative stress levels many patients had, and I worried about food grown in soils depleted of minerals.

· ·

THE MAPS OF THE U.S. SHOWING THE OBESITY RATES DECADE BY DECADE TOOK MY BREATH AWAY.

· ·

I was surprised when Dr. Servan-Schreiber said he agreed with me. I don't know why I was surprised though. How could I have imagined that such an accomplished physician and scientist, and authority on lifestyle and cancer, was not aware of such things?

Dr. Servan-Schreiber admitted that he had avoided such discussions in his book for one reason: fear of censure from the medical community. I was surprised at that as well.

Dr. Servan-Schreiber's lecture during "Cancer Guides II" was as amazing as his book. He spent a lot of time showing how agriculture and the American food supply chain have changed over the decades. A large focus was on the shift, decades ago, to change some of the food given to livestock, a change from grass to grain. Grass, or pasture, contains beneficial omega-3 fatty acids, and beef from cattle grazing on grass contains the same beneficial fatty acids as does wild salmon.

Although almost all cattle are raised on pasture, seldom are they "grass-finished." Over the last few decades, cattle are no longer slaughtered at the end of a long day of grazing. Instead, for the last three weeks of life, most beef cattle are penned up in a feedlot and stuffed with corn and soy. These "grain-finished" cattle gain huge amounts of weight quickly. This is good for the financial bottom line, as cattle are sold by weight.

Dr. Servan-Schreiber went on to explain how corn oil and soybean oil are very inflammatory, full of omega-6 fatty acids. These inflammatory fatty acids accumulate in the flesh of cows feeding in grains containing these oils. When humans ingest beef full of these inflammatory oils, heart disease, diabetes, and cancer ensue. Over the last 50 years, Americans have consumed more and more grain-fed meat, which may contribute to an increase in disease, including cancer.

The maps of the U.S. showing the obesity rates decade by decade took my breath away. The trajectory stunned me, because I knew that obesity was linked to many types of cancer. Dr. Servan-Schreiber went on to illustrate how cancer rates have climbed in wealthy countries. Even in Japan, where cancer rates have historically been quite low—often attributed to the traditional Japanese diet containing lots of vegetables and soy—cancer has been on the rise for years.

The lecture ended and left me full of disturbing thoughts.

Dr. Servan-Schreiber's book, *Anticancer*, would became a *New York Times* Best Seller. It has been translated into 35 languages, with over one million copies in print. Dr. Servan-Schreiber dedicated the last years of his life to educating the public about a sensible integrative approach to cancer care through audio books, lectures and seminars.

I would run into Dr. Servan-Schreiber only once more, at the Society for Integrative Oncology conference that would be held in November 2010. We would both be ill at that meeting, he more so than I. Dr. Servan-Schreiber died in July 2011, not long after our last meeting.

But during "Cancer Guides II" in June 2009, I felt fine. After Dr. Servan-Schreiber's lecture, I attended the talk by Devra Davis, PhD, MPH, an epidemiologist from the University of Pittsburgh, and founding director of the Center for Environmental Oncology. She spoke on the relationship between environmental pollutants and cancer, things like the chemical load used in conventional dry cleaning, the possible dangers of cellular phone transmission, and the toxicity of thermal paper used in cash register receipts. What an informative, but scary, session hers was.

Another lecture that I found fascinating was given by Dieter Hager, MD, PhD, a European medical scientist, clinician, and pioneer in the use of mistletoe extract and hyperthermia in cancer treatment. Both of these therapeutic approaches were new to me. The theory behind hyperthermia is that heating the body increases the effectiveness of chemotherapy and radiation. Both mistletoe and hyperthermia treatments are available in Europe. However, in the United States, mistletoe is still considered an investigational drug, and hyperthermia treatment is not covered by most health insurance policies.

I also met with Ralph Moss, PhD, who for several decades has chronicled the evolution of integrative cancer therapies. A patient advocate and coach, known as a sharp critic of what some call "The Cancer Establishment," he publishes *The Moss Reports*. These comprehensive monographs on conventional and non-conventional approaches to many cancers have proven invaluable to countless patients.

One of the few speakers I had not emailed was Jeffery White, MD, who was—and still is—Director of the National Institutes of Health's Office of Cancer Complementary and Alternative Medicine (OCCAM). As Dr. White gave his presentation, discussing OCCAM's role (and thus, his role) in funding integrative oncology research, I realized what a mistake I'd made by not contacting him before the conference.

As soon as Dr. White finished speaking, I practically sprinted to the podium. Unfortunately for me, someone else beat me to him. I waited anxiously until that conversation was finished. Then I started to introduce myself. I had barely gushed out my name when Dr. White interrupted. "I know exactly who you are."

My heart sank. I thought he was going to give me the brush-off. Instead, he turned and hurried for the door, but motioned me to follow. He was talking. I had to speed up to get close enough to hear.

Dr. White told me that he had already spoken to Dr. Rosenthal, knew my story, and thought I really ought to apply for funding. My jaw dropped.

From what I understood, funding a study on the effects of vegetables, vitamins and exercise on patients with chronic lymphocytic leukemia had not been part of the NIH's plan. Apparently detecting my shock, Dr. White explained that whether the application for funding was approved would ultimately be for the reviewers to decide. But in his opinion, I ought to give it a try.

He strode out of the conference, leaving me feeling as charged as I had ever felt. My dream was coming true. My n-of-1 experiment had caught the attention of "the scientific medical establishment." I had little time to celebrate however. I had to hurry back to the conference hall. One of the next speakers was Dr. Keith Block. 🌱

58

I WAS SITTING RESTLESSLY in the conference room trying, in vain, to pay attention to the speaker. But my mind kept traveling to my business emails about selling the company until, out of the corner of my eye, I spied a tall man dressed in a suit and tie, who had risen from his seat near the front. I recognized the dark hair and intense eyes from photos on the internet. It was Dr. Keith Block.

Dr. Block was scheduled to speak next. But instead of walking to the podium, Dr. Block was edging down the side aisle toward the back of the conference hall. My chance had arrived! On a quest, I slipped from my seat as well. Imagine my chagrin when, after following him out of the conference hall, I realized he was heading for the restroom!

I felt a little sheepish for practically stalking the guy. But I was desperate. Despite the email exchange promising a meeting, I had not had an opportunity to approach him and set it up.

He pushed through the swinging door to the men's room. I hesitated. But only for a moment. Shameless, I pushed through the door right after him.

I waited as discreetly as I could. When the moment was right, I pounced. "I'm Glenn Sabin," I said, extending my just-washed hand.

"Ah yes," Dr. Block responded, shaking my hand. "You have leukemia. Let's try to talk before the conference ends." With that, he headed back to the conference hall and took the podium.

Dr. Block is a residency-trained internist who studied nutritional oncology and has dedicated his career to cancer treatment. He is the founding editor of the journal *Integrative Cancer Therapies*, and was instrumental in launching integrative medicine education for medical students at the University of Illinois at Chicago. Together with his wife Dr. Penny Block, a specialist in psycho-oncology and biobehavioral oncology, Dr. Keith Block founded the Block Center for Integrative Cancer Treatment. At this facility, since 1980, the Blocks have combined conventional treatments with integrative modalities such as chronomodulated chemotherapy and targeted supplements, as well as diet, exercise, and stress reduction techniques.

That day at the conference, Dr. Block's talk covered the three core tenets of the Block Center's model of integrative cancer care: biography, biology, and pathology.

"Biography" takes into account who the patient is, and how they live. This includes not only food choices and exercise habits, but the emotional tone of a person's days. Is the person harried, hassled, or hostile? Or easygoing? "Biography" also includes an accounting of major events in a patient's health, social, and psychological history. All of these aspects are examined to pinpoint areas for intervention.

· ·

**DR. BLOCK ALSO PRESENTED AN IDEA
NEW TO ME, THE IDEA OF THE TUMOR
"MICROENVIRONMENT."**

· ·

The next core area, "Biology," refers to the state of a patient's ability to resist disease, or the patient's "terrain." Block uses various blood test panels such as those that quantify all of the following: nutrient levels, inflammation, blood sugar levels, oxidative stress (free radicals), and stress hormones.

Dr. Block recommends that the terrain be repeatedly measured and attended to, in order to maximize a patient's chance of recovery. This is because abnormal inflammatory responses and oxidative stress can promote the growth of cancer, and because cancer itself can increase inflammation and oxidative stress; thus a deleterious loop is set in motion.

In addition, Dr. Block believes that cancer treatment, such as surgery, chemotherapy, and radiation, and a patient's metabolic problems such as high blood sugar and insulin levels, can also drive cancer growth, and this effect needs to be mitigated.

Pathology, the third core area, refers to the cancer itself. Dr. Block emphasized that his approach to treating cancer uses conventional treatments. However, his approach differs from conventional oncology practices because a comprehensive system that combines diet, physical care, psychological care, and nutraceuticals is central to the practice. By lessening the side effects of conventional therapies, especially chemotherapy, this approach, Dr. Block hypothesizes, results in fewer treatment delays, allows reduction of drug doses, and increases the body's innate ability to resist tumor growth.

Dr. Block touched on other aspects of his program, on exercise (at the Block Center patients gently ride exercise bicycles while receiving chemotherapy infusions), on circadian rhythms, restorative sleep, strategies to deal with emotional stress, and on the importance of a strong social and psychological support network.

Dr. Block also presented an idea new to me, the idea of the tumor "microenvironment."

Surrounding and within a cancerous tumor are many normal cells. Two types of normal cells in this so-called "tumor microenvironment" are especially prone to hijacking: those cells forming blood vessel walls, and those belonging to the immune system.

Cancerous cells communicate with their normal neighbors by sending out chemical messages (as do normal cells). Specifically, cancer cells release chemical requests for a blood supply and for immune protection. With Block's explanation, I could understand why a cancerous tumor would want a good blood supply.

What surprised me even more is how a cancerous tumor hijacks healthy immune cells, reprograms them to protect the cancer, and sets them on sentry duty in the tumor microenvironment. It's these hijacked immune cells that provide the tumor with protection from the larger immune system.

Block's explanation of how the ability of normal immune cells to resist these hijack attempts is weakened by an unhealthy lifestyle—a sugar-laden diet, lack of exercise, missed sleep, and unrelieved stress—made perfect sense to me. The good news was that a body well cared for is more likely to deny the tumor's demands for support. This built-in cancer resistance is exactly what Dr. Block's program aims to enhance.

The program I had cobbled together over the years was nearly as complex as the one Dr. Block recommended, and I was proud of my efforts. But in all my work with supplements, I had never measured the vitamin and mineral levels in my blood, let alone measured my inflammatory markers. In contrast, Dr. Block routinely performed comprehensive lab tests at least every four months. These included saliva tests for levels of the stress hormone cortisol and the hormone melatonin, which mediates sleep onset. Dr. Block used the results to inform a range of both food-based and nutraceutical interventions, ones that he believed would help patients maintain an internal "anticancer terrain."

This approach made sense to me. Why not use blood tests to determine my specific needs, and then tailor my nutraceutical program exactly?

The lecture ended. As I joined in the applause, I recalled seeing Dr. Block's book, *Life Over Cancer*, for sale on a table just outside the meeting room. I figured that after such a great talk, the several dozen copies would sell out quickly, so I hurried out to grab a copy. Subsequently I would ask him sign it, and get to really meet him that way. That was the plan.

A few minutes later, with book in hand, I returned to the meeting hall and headed toward the podium. But there were so many people crowding Dr. Block that I was only able to squeeze in a "Thanks for a great talk." Not the meeting I had hoped for.

Finally, late that afternoon I cornered him again, just outside the lecture hall. Desperate to set up a private meeting before I lost him to the crowd, I quickly blurted out my story and my interest in meeting with him.

Dr. Block agreed to reconnect with me, but only after I had read *Life Over Cancer*. Maybe he thought the intricacies of his program would scare me off. If so, he was wrong. I had already decided that I wanted him to be my next mentor.

Now, at the time of that conference in June 2009, although I was under terrible stress from the sale of my family's business, I felt entirely well. I had no idea that I would soon need Dr. Block not as a mentor, but as a physician. 🍷

59

THE FIRST TIME I VISITED THE BLOCK CENTER in Evanston, Illinois was September 4, 2009. I pushed open the double glass doors to find myself in a high-ceilinged lobby, awash in serene colors. The sounds of flowing water and birdsong soothed me, and a nature scene unfolded on a large plasma wall monitor.

Something else caught my interest. Through a glass wall, I saw a fully decked-out kitchen, and someone busily cooking! There were people standing around watching, some of them tethered to rolling IV poles. I went to the kitchen door and let myself in. A dietician-chef was demonstrating how to prepare a healthy meal to a half dozen people. The chef discussed all of the ingredients, and had those items in plain sight for all to see the brand name and packaging.

Although I had been in many medical institutions in the eighteen years since my diagnosis, I'd never seen anything like this! As I pondered that fact, the center's research manager, Dr. Charlotte Gyllenhaal, came to retrieve me. She was going to give me a tour of the facility. I had already gotten a feel for the center, and was very impressed. There were more wonders ahead.

In her 30-year career at the University of Illinois, Charlotte Gyllenhaal, PhD, traveled the world seeking medicinal plants. Countless drugs are derived from plants, and many of them are used to fight cancer: vinorelbine, vincristine, taxol, and taxotere, to name but a few.

Every room in the Block Center was named after a plant, and I wondered if Dr. Gyllenhall had had something to do with that. As she was pointing out the names, I noted that a mezuzah, (a prayer on a scroll in a metal container), graced each doorway. I hadn't realized how comforting this homage to my heritage would be.

Following Dr. Gyllenhaal down a hallway, I poked my head into an empty exam room. The walls, the paintings, even the careful arrangement of the furniture, somehow exuded calm. It was as though every detail of the physical space had been crafted to elicit serenity, and a sense of connection to nature. Nothing about the place resembled the hospitals, centers and clinics I had visited in the past.

The tour ended with Dr. Gyllenhaal depositing me back at the kitchen. The chef was just wrapping up the cooking demonstration, and I was presented with a wonderful plate of salmon and a fresh, colorful array of veggies.

Then it was time to meet with Dr. Block. He came in with his colleague and wife Penny Block, cofounder and executive director of the clinic. She earned a PhD in psychosocial oncology from the University of Chicago. Dr. Penny Block was in charge of training the Center's integrative staff, and of overseeing the mind-body and biobehavioral aspects of the clinic's program.

· ·

THAT WAS WHEN DR. NADLER GAVE ME
THE SHOCKING NEWS.

· ·

In the three months that had passed since the "Cancer Guides II" conference, I had read *Life Over Cancer*, not once but twice, soaking up its wisdom. Both times I was amazed at how closely the Block Center's program aligned with my experience. I was well prepared for my first meeting with Dr. Block.

I knew that Dr. Block believed that the effectiveness of conventional treatments could be enhanced by a plant-based diet with moderate amounts of cold water fish, stress control techniques, regular exercise, restorative sleep, and judicious supplement use, guided by frequent blood tests.

I had been looking forward to this meeting for months. By the time I finally sat down with Dr. Block, I was determined to tell him everything I could about my approach to dealing with my diagnosis. I was confident he would be interested in my story, and it was important to me to get his input.

I talked with Dr. Block, and reviewed the nutraceuticals I had taken over the years, emphasizing the ones I believed had helped me recover from the acute CLL flare-up in 2003. He was intrigued by my narrative. I felt we were closely aligned philosophically. By the time we parted late in the afternoon, my connection with Dr. Block and his approach was confirmed. I had my new mentor.

I had considered that first visit to the Block Center purely educational, part of my FON-related duties to make connections with leaders in integrative oncology. I thoroughly enjoyed the initial visit to the Block Clinic. Who wouldn't? After all, it was a beautiful facility, and I felt that Dr. Block was a brilliant thinker, and perhaps most importantly, I hadn't gone as a patient. In the six years since I had last successfully pushed back against leukemia, I had felt perfectly well.

Barely a month after my meeting with Dr. Block, I went to Dana-Farber for a routine checkup. That was when Dr. Nadler gave me the shocking news.

The leukemia was no longer in remission. ❦

60

MY WHITE BLOOD CELL COUNT was abnormally high, at around 14,700 cells per microliter. Not only that, my red blood cells were slightly low, and my absolute lymphocyte count was elevated. The leukemia was once again active.

This change of events was no surprise to Dr. Nadler. He had been expecting it, and he was not particularly worried. He assured me that a long time, months, perhaps years, might pass before I needed treatment. All we needed to do at that very time was measure the white count every few months, and note how long it took to double. The longer the doubling time, the better the chances of avoiding treatment, at least for a while. "Don't worry about it," he told me.

Of course, not worrying about something like advancing cancer is impossible. I worried and ruminated endlessly, turning over and over everything that had transpired in my life. What had happened, what had I done wrong?

It was November 2009. Over the years, I had kept up with all aspects of my program: diet, exercise, sleep, and supplements. So, what had changed? Then I hit upon something. Stress. The six-month period preceding the sale of my company in July 2009 had been brutal. Was I now paying with my health?

I had considered myself immune to such things. But now I wondered if I had been deluding myself. I had gone through an enormously stressful period. Day in and day out, the problems kept coming without a break. Why would I consider that to be a problem for others, but not for me?

Like most people, I have to work for a living. I have to deal with the everyday pressures of life, marriage, family, and finances. As it turned out, I wasn't immune. It seemed that the relentlessness of the last round of stress had finally gotten to me. ♥

• PART IV •

MISSION POSSIBLE

61

SHORTLY AFTER I GOT THE NEWS about my latest relapse, I attended the 2009 Society for Integrative Oncology (SIO) conference in Manhattan.

One of the keynote speakers was Dr. Dean Ornish. He is founder and president of the Preventive Medicine Research Institute (PMRI) in Sausalito, California, and a clinical professor of medicine at the University of California, San Francisco. To me, he is also an absolute rock star of lifestyle medicine. Dr. Ornish spent his early career demonstrating that diet, exercise, and stress reduction can reverse "irreversible" heart disease. Before 1990, when Dr. Ornish began publishing his findings, doctors believed that the best option for patients with severely clogged coronary arteries was bypass surgery, a dangerous, debilitating, and expensive procedure. Then Dr. Ornish came along with a very different approach: he cleaned out arteries with vegetables, meditation, social support, and long walks. Adoption of his recommendations took almost two decades, and then the cardiology community was, by 2009, routinely prescribing such lifestyle changes for heart attack patients.

With that matter having been addressed, Dr. Ornish turned his attention to cancer. At the time of the conference, Dr. Ornish was in the midst of the first randomized controlled trial that showed that comprehensive lifestyle changes may halt, or even reverse, the progression of early-stage prostate cancer. The set of interventions he used included a near-vegan diet, supplemental selenium, lycopene, and vitamin E, stress reduction, and moderate exercise. Dr. Ornish went on to show that these comprehensive lifestyle changes affect gene expression, the "turning on" and "turning off" of genes that prevent or promote cancer.

Dr. Ornish's work on the key role of lifestyle in heart disease and prostate cancer is incredibly important and instructive, and its acceptance into practice came to fruition over tall odds. His accomplishments should have inspired me. But I barely heard a word of his keynote presentation. I was too distracted by a terrible fact. Once again, I was fighting for my life. ♥

62

IT WAS DEEP IN THE AUTUMN OF 2009 when I returned to the Block Center, this time as a patient. What stands out in my memory of that day is the crunch of snow underfoot, and a wind so cold it made my face ache.

I was nonetheless grateful. I know this may sound strange, but I was excited to be in the Chicago area, and eager to be at the Block Center as a patient. In fact, I was almost elated. I'd long been very impressed with the man and his work. Now I was about to experience this groundbreaking clinic from the patient's perspective. I don't mean to make light of this decision. I had been working with Rosenberg for 10 years, and he was incredibly helpful during my acute episode in 2003. However, this new relapse made it obvious that the nutraceutical program was no longer working. The rising white blood counts made that very clear.

By the time I arrived at the Block Center, my white blood counts had climbed again, from 14,000 to 17,000, and the hemoglobin and hematocrit were still dropping. I was in trouble. It was time to make another move.

Even though the Block Center employed several oncologists, I did not see any of them. There was no need for that, because I was seen regularly by Dr. Kressel. Nonetheless, I had a full schedule that day. I met with an internist, a registered dietician, and finally with Dr. Block. It felt like an inordinate amount of time and attention. And it was. In fact, my first visit to the Block Center lasted five hours. The relaxed pace was new to me, and wonderful.

Dr. Block ordered blood tests to evaluate oxidative stress, immune function, insulin production, inflammation, vitamin and mineral levels, toxins, even the antioxidant capacity and viscosity of my blood. Saliva tests would measure cortisol and melatonin levels.

I had been taking a large array and volume of nutraceuticals over an 18-year period, with little feedback, no way of knowing what, if anything, was being accomplished. Now with these additional blood tests, I would be moving things to a whole new level. Dr. Block assured me that any deficits in my health regimen would become glaringly evident when I received the test results.

Oddly, I almost looked forward to learning what those problems might be. I found it comforting to know that abnormalities in my blood work could tell me how to improve the diet, exercise, and supplement choices I made every day. 🍃

63

MY LAB REPORTS CAME BACK looking pretty good overall, but there was work to be done. My essential fatty acid ratio between omega 3 and 6 was about 1:3, where Dr. Block wanted to see 1:2 or even 1:1. Omega 3 fatty acids are the ones famously contained in wild salmon and other cold-water fish.

Dr. Block worried that inflammation might drive the growth of my leukemia cells. My inflammatory markers were fairly low, but he wanted them lower. Dairy products can increase inflammation, and I am a guy that if left to my own, could have pizza twice a day. At that point I was averaging one cheese pizza with Miles and Jared every month or so. That brings to mind the time I met the Blocks in D.C. for dinner. I ordered a Caesar salad, complete with parmesan cheese. As I tucked into it, I noted a single raised eyebrow from Dr. Block. Thereafter, I cut dairy back to almost nothing!

Vitamin D is incredibly important for so many aspects of health and prevention. Although my blood serum level of vitamin D was 47 ng/ml, in the normal range, Dr. Block wanted it higher. Additional food recommendations were made, and other compounds were added to my diet, to help increase the absorption rate. There was concern in case I had a genetic make-up that predisposed me to difficulties with vitamin D processing, which may have been underlying the level at the low end of the normal range. Over a few months, we elevated the level to 74 ng/ml. Today my vitamin D level hovers right under 90 ng/ml, and I monitor it regularly with the rest of my blood work. When necessary, I adjust my dose of vitamin D to keep the level consistent.

Because a high insulin level is thought to encourage the growth of many cancers, Dr. Block wanted my insulin level to be as low as possible. The pancreas secretes insulin when carbohydrates are ingested, and an elevated level of C-peptide on a blood test reveals that excess insulin has been secreted. I do have a minor sweet tooth, so I was not surprised that at first, my C-peptide level was on the high side.

Dr. Block urged me to cut down further on sweets. So I began diluting my fruit juices, replacing half with water. On Dr. Block's advice, I also increased the amount of lipoic acid and other antioxidant supplements I was taking, as he believed this would help decrease the C-peptide level. All of this seemed to help, because the follow up C-peptide test improved nicely.

D-dimer is a marker of blood coagulation, which is involved in cancer spread, and therefore Dr. Block wanted mine low. But mine was sky high. A few months of supplemental curcumin, fish oil, and the herb scutellaria, and my d-dimer level plummeted to near normal.

Another marker of coagulation, the prothrombin fragments test, started out markedly high. Fortunately, as I adhered to my new supplement regimen, this coagulation marker also dropped to a normal level.

Dr. Block also recommended that I started a supplement containing green tea and reishi mushroom, both for their known anticancer activity.

This entire regimen would eventually decrease my inflammatory markers to a wonderfully low level.

The way I have written this, it may sound as if I started the recommendations right away. Even with such a stellar physician on my side, I was ever the skeptic. Before doing something to my body, I insisted on doing my own research, and I had to be sure I agreed with Dr. Block's advice. It wouldn't be until May 2010 that I started on my new Block Center nutraceutical program.

I soon ran into another obstacle. I found myself taking nearly 70 pills a day. 🍂

64

IT WAS LINDA'S MOM COOKIE who came to the rescue and organized my new pill regimen. This wasn't the first time I had taken lots of pills. After being diagnosed with leukemia, I had taken numerous supplements, sometimes dozens daily, and always under supervision. Three times a year, for many years running, Linda's mom Cookie would come over to the house and set up a little production line on our dining room table. There she would assemble four months' worth of supplement packets. The project required several hours, scores of cups, many bottles of supplements, and numerous small resealable plastic bags. At the end of the production line would be rows of my daily packets of pills, all impeccably organized in their little plastic bags.

Cookie's labor spared me having to open a dozen or so bottles a couple of times per day, and then dispensing specific amounts of pills. The packets also made travel a breeze. I just threw the needed number of packets into my luggage. Linda and I still do it this way today. With the tremendous number of pills I now had to take, Cookie's help was even more invaluable.

As for the supplement program, I couldn't say as much.

Despite adhering to Dr. Block's supplement regimen for six months, by October 2010, my total white blood cell count measured a whopping 47,000. Not only that, the anemia was worsening. In fact, almost every blood count was now abnormal.

I felt fine. But my blood counts told me that I was getting sicker. 🍇

65

IT WAS LATE 2010, and in response to these worsening blood results, Dr. Block increased the amount of epigallocatechin-3-gallate, (EGCG), in my regimen. This was the same green tea component I'd heard about in 2005, when it was being studied by Dr. Kay at the Mayo Clinic in Minnesota. Dr. Kay's studies had shown that some CLL patients improved with high doses of EGCG, and based on this evidence, Dr. Block decided that a higher dose was worth a try for me.

But over the next few months, my white count continued to rise. On February 11, 2011 it was over 50,000. To say I was discouraged would be an understatement. ♥

66

BY MARCH 2011, my white blood cell count began to drop. At 30 thousand, it was still high, no doubt about it. But for the first time in a year, there was some improvement.

I tried not to hope for much. How could I stand the disappointment? I reminded myself that this was a small and possibly questionable improvement. It might even have been a fluke, certainly no cause for a big celebration. But in my heart of hearts, I hoped.

Because maybe—just maybe—this was the tiny beginning to a big turnaround. And I secretly asked myself a question I probably should not have asked.

EGCG. Was it working? 🍃

67

AT ABOUT THAT TIME, Dr. Nadler's office called and told me that Dr. Nadler wanted to see me in clinic. It was a fair request; after all, at the very beginning I had asked him to monitor my condition. But I wasn't ready to see him. My new improvement felt fragile, and I needed to wait until I was sure the leukemia was coming under control.

I emailed Dr. Nadler to let him know that I was working with a new integrative medicine physician, and I felt we were on the right track with our approach. Dr. Nadler emailed back, asking that I keep him updated on my blood test results and he urged me to schedule an appointment with him soon. Still, I couldn't bring myself to do it.

Given that I felt perfectly well during this period, I continued full steam ahead on every aspect of my lifestyle regimen. By the end of May 2011, my white blood cells had decreased to 19,000. Although this value was still well over the normal level, this was a clear and major improvement. Other blood tests' values were also improving.

With a little more confidence that I was on the right track with my regimen, I emailed Dr. Nadler. Although, I still wasn't ready to make an appointment, I was a bit cocky about my improved blood counts. I told him that I was sure the nutraceutical mix I was on was working. "See you in clinic," I wrote, "once I put my body into clinical remission, *again*!"

He did not respond.

By mid-July my white blood cell count had fallen to 9,400, which was within the normal range. By November 2011, about a year after increasing the dose of EGCG, my white blood cell count was 5,600, at the low end of normal! In addition to the dramatic decrease in my white blood cells, every single number in my terrain report had returned to within the normal range. A complete blood count and flow cytometry of the blood found no CLL cells. My blood was normal.

I was in clinical remission. Again. The feeling of turning back the tide of the leukemia for a second time, albeit from a less acute episode, was exhilarating.

I had recovered from the effects of full-blown leukemia in 2003, when I was working with Irv Rosenberg. At that time, Dr. Nadler hadn't wanted to do a marrow biopsy because he was afraid the disappointment of finding out I still had leukemia would damage my spirit. It was Dr. Kressel who ended up doing the bone marrow biopsy, and it had shown that my marrow still contained leukemia cells.

Now in 2011, I was working with Dr. Block. I had tried a powerful new program, which, among other things, contained EGCG. My response had been spectacular. I had a strange thought. Not only was I feeling well, I had good blood counts. Was my bone marrow free of leukemic cells?

I wanted to find out. I wanted another bone marrow biopsy. This time I wanted it done by Dr. Nadler, at Harvard. I wanted one of the world's most well-regarded and conservative medical institutions to document my results. ♥

68

IN NOVEMBER 2011, I emailed Dr. Nadler to tell him all that had happened. I attached all my lab reports, showing the inexorable improvement, and finally, normal blood test results. I told him I was ready to see him in clinic and undergo the usual tests, all except the PET/CT. In the email, I also asked Dr. Nadler if he would do a bone marrow biopsy. I wanted this test to see if my bone marrow had cleared.

I waited a couple of weeks but did not get a response. I doubted if Dr. Nadler was avoiding me; after all, he had given me his private cell phone number in years past. Finally I called him on that cell phone. When we spoke, I made it clear to him that I was a bit peeved that he hadn't responded to my email. He buttered me up a bit, telling me I was his smartest patient, and that what I had accomplished was amazing. I fell for the compliments, hook, line and sinker.

Dr. Nadler then pressed me to undergo the PET/CT, saying it was the standard way to detect lymph node enlargement in CLL. I strongly resisted this idea. In all the years since my diagnosis, I'd never had any swollen lymph nodes. In my opinion, a PET/CT wasn't worth the risk of a secondary, radiation-induced, cancer down the road. Dr. Nadler acquiesced: no PET/CT.

He discouraged a bone marrow biopsy. And I think I understood his position. After all, he had been correct in 2003, when he told me that a bone marrow biopsy that showed persistent leukemia might spoil my happiness at achieving a clinical remission. Indeed it had. Yet I'd survived the disappointment, and not only that, I'd survived much worse.

Now in November 2011, I really wanted another bone marrow biopsy, and I explained to Dr. Nader in detail, the reasons why. I was willing to risk another disappointment to learn the truth. My expectations were in check, and I was well aware that there were no reports of any patient having successfully cleared their marrow of CLL without chemotherapy or radiation. Furthermore, even those modalities usually failed to clear the marrow. So, I knew that it was extremely unlikely that the new biopsy would show that I had a "clean" marrow, one free of leukemia cells. I was completely prepared for that result. But, being Glenn Sabin the fledgling investigator, I needed to see if that expectation was wrong.

Dr. Nadler was silent. I felt a little sheepish. After all, I had called him on his private cell line, interrupting who knows what, and then proceeded to tell him that

I, a credential-free layman-on-a-mission, disagreed with his experienced and expert opinion. I was asking him to help me obtain testing that wasn't clinically necessary.

In Dr. Nadler's decades of caring for CLL patients, not once had a patient cleared his or her marrow of leukemia while pursuing only a lifestyle program. Was there any reason to think I was outside that group?

· ·

I, A CREDENTIAL-FREE LAYMAN-ON-A-MISSION, DIS-AGREED WITH HIS EXPERIENCED AND EXPERT OPINION.

· ·

There was, at least to my mind. I had tried something novel. I had carried out my lifestyle changes in as organized a way as I knew how. And it seemed to have worked. In fact, it seemed to have worked far better than anyone had expected. So I kept talking.

The chance I was onto something was indeed small, I said, and I understood that. But not examining the marrow again now, when I was well, would be bad science; no one would know if there was a relationship between how I was feeling, and what was happening in my bone marrow. The n-of-1 experiment with Glenn Sabin would have a critical data point missing!

I told Dr. Nadler that I was determined to have a bone marrow biopsy, and that I would prefer that he do it, because I wanted to have the best pathologists in the world review my marrow. But if he was not able to do the procedure, I was prepared to get it done elsewhere, because it was going to get done. I was completely insufferable!

Unlike me, Dr. Nadler was always a gentleman, and was helpful whenever possible. Or perhaps on that occasion he just wanted to shut me up? By the end of the phone call, he had agreed to my request, and would do the bone marrow biopsy for me. A few hours later I was lying prone in his office, the long biopsy needle poised above the back of my hipbone.

Then it was done, and I went home to pass the week before the bone marrow biopsy results would be available. 💙

69

THE WEEK OF WAITING PASSED QUICKLY. But once it had, whenever I would pick up the phone to call Dr. Nadler's office to get the results, the disappointment of the 2003 report would become raw again, and I would hang up even before the first ring. Then I would curse.

Dr. Nadler had been right in 2003, and he was right again in 2011. Waiting for the results of the bone marrow biopsy was making a wreck out of me. Between attempted phone calls, I berated myself. Demanding a bone marrow biopsy! How stupid was that? It appeared that I had put the CLL into clinical remission, and instead of savoring my accomplishment, I'd insisted on viewing the whole thing as a scientific experiment. I was being ridiculous. How could I separate Glenn-the-research-subject from Glenn-the-patient? Was I asking too much of supplements, green tea and a thoughtfully constructed diet and lifestyle? Was a clean marrow too much to hope for?

Probably.

The trouble was, I couldn't stop myself from hoping.

A few weeks after the biopsy, an envelope arrived. I knew there would be two documents inside, Dr. Nadler's clinical report and a pathology report. Although I was a moment away from getting the results I'd begged for, I froze. ❦

70

THERE WERE ONLY TWO POSSIBLE OUTCOMES of my marrow biopsy: leukemic cells were either present or they were absent. This sounds so simple. It was anything but.

According to the medical literature, and in the personal experience of my oncologists, no CLL patient had ever cleared leukemic cells from their bone marrow with vegetables, filtered water, exercise, and supplements. So it was unlikely I had accomplished that feat. It would hardly be news if I had leukemic cells in my marrow. Nor would it be failure. For almost 20 years I had had leukemic cells in my marrow. Not only was I quite alive, I was healthier now than I'd been as a young man!

All this logic did nothing to quiet the thumping in my chest as I stared at the two documents. Which should I read first? Dr. Nadler's clinical report, or the pathology report?

By now I pretty much knew what to expect from Dr. Nadler's clinical report. These notes were in standard medical format. They always started by cataloging my recent symptoms (or lack thereof), and what medications and supplements I'd been taking. Next came a review of the physical examination and listing of test results. Last came Dr. Nadler's opinion about the state of my health, and an outline of the next steps to be taken.

It was the pathology report, the second document, which contained the results of the bone marrow biopsy. I simply couldn't bear to read it.

I couldn't live without reading it.

I smoothed out the creases and began to read. ❦

71

AS I SCANNED THE REPORT, a chill shot up my spine. Was I reading it accurately? Was it saying what I thought it was saying?

"Flow cytometric study of bone marrow and peripheral blood do not reveal diagnostic features of involvement by a lymphoproliferative disorder. Overall, definitive diagnostic features of involvement by a B cell lymphoproliferative disorder are not seen. (Clinical: 48 year old male with history of chronic lymphocytic leukemia with no prior medical treatment.)"

It took me a moment to translate these sentences from medical-ese to English. The two most important words were *not seen*. What exactly was *not seen?* Leukemia. *There was no sign that I had ever had it.* My marrow was stone cold normal.

I could not wrap my mind around this astonishing fact. The report seemed to be saying that the leukemia, the disease that had defined my life for 20 years, was gone. Could that be? Was the report in error? Was I missing something? I fumbled for the phone. I dialed Dr. Nadler's cell phone number. He answered immediately. ❧

72

DR. NADLER WAS ASTONISHED. There was no leukemia in my marrow. I was in full clinical remission. I might even be cured.

Cured.

These wonderful results occurred without conventional treatment. I was already focusing on my next steps. How I could share this lifestyle choice and whole person approach with other people. Where would I start?

Dr. Nadler suggested looking into EGCG. But I reminded him that not all patients in the Mayo Clinic trials enjoyed a robust response to EGCG.

Could it be the other lifestyle and supplement interventions had also helped? Was synergy between several factors at work? Rather than one component of my program, such as EGCG, being entirely responsible for my recovery, was it possible that the various elements of my program had worked together to improve my health?

I recall Dr. Nadler countering that whether a patient responded to EGCG might not be related to lifestyle interventions. Instead it might be related to immunoglobulin levels, or perhaps be related to genetic patterns in the leukemic cells, patterns that would almost certainly differ from patient to patient.

But what about the fact that I had recovered from CLL related anemia at the end of 2003 without any EGCG? I had been exercising, drinking pure water, minding my stress, and eating gorgeous produce free of pesticides. And my supplement regimen was quite different at that time.

Our discussion continued along these lines, until I had a realization: Dr. Nadler and I were in the same church, but in different pews.

I wasn't sure what he was getting at, but I wondered if he thought that EGCG alone was responsible for the remission. To my mind, that was one possible answer. However, what if synergy was involved? That was another possible answer. There were probably more possibilities. Getting as many answers as I could would occupy me for several years

There would, however, always be more questions. But for now, I savored these three sweet words: full pathological remission. 🌱

EPILOGUE

CLL, LIKE MOST CANCERS, REMAINS AN ENIGMA. Conventional medicine is making great strides, but still cannot offer a cure. However, integrative medicine has done well by me. As of this writing in late 2015 I remain well. My most recent blood tests, including flow cytometry, could find no evidence that I've ever had CLL. Only time will tell if I am truly cured.

But however things go, I know now that I am not at the mercy of CLL, or of any disease. Nor do I have to accept at face value the limited understanding of the good doctors who have dedicated their lives to understanding CLL. I am very prepared to help myself. With the support of my doctors, Kressel, Nadler and Block, and my mentors Pelton and Rosenberg, and with my incredible wife Linda helping me, I will search for effective ways to meet leukemia, should it recur.

As my story spreads, I have been invited to speak at scientific and health conferences aimed at cancer patients and physicians. My purpose in accepting these invitations is to give hope to those struggling with cancer or other potentially deadly conditions, to open their minds to the idea that there may be much they can do for themselves to heal. I tell audiences that for me, lifestyle choices were powerful, the benefits exceeding the probable outcomes of offered chemotherapy. And I hope to reach physicians, to let them know that for me, lifestyle interventions appeared to accomplish what conventional treatment could not.

I understand that what worked for me will not work for everyone. And I do understand that association is not causation. In other words, perhaps the interventions I made were not responsible for my remarkable recovery. Perhaps some other event I am unaware of, or some inherent characteristic of my particular condition, was responsible for my exceptional recovery.

And for that reason, I don't encourage anyone to eschew conventional treatment. Nor should anyone copy my diet or supplement protocols. That would be foolish, as they were designed for me alone. Instead, I want every cancer patient to get the help they need to work out their own successful protocols, tailored to their unique health needs.

In closing, I call on conventional physicians and investigators to put serious resources to work looking into cases like mine, where an unexpected recovery occurs. Please, conduct the rigorous research needed to learn how best to use diet, exercise, stress reduction techniques, herbs, and supplements to help people with serious illness. The time is now for this approach to become a major thrust of research.

Finally, I call on patients and their loved ones to support the doctors on the front lines of this approach: integrative physicians.

. . . .

SO WHY HAVE DECADES OF LARGE STUDIES LEFT US WITHOUT CURES FOR CANCER?

. . . .

Over these last years, I have had the privilege of interacting with many leading physicians and scientists working to advance integrative medicine. Thanks to these pioneers, medical research no longer centers solely on supposedly homogenous groups of patients who undergo an identical treatment.

The large, randomized, double-blind, placebo-controlled trial was a godsend in its early days, when it proved a powerful tool for finding cures for many infectious diseases. So why have decades of large studies left us without cures for cancer?

It's not the fault of the study design. Despite having powerful tools that minimize bias—randomization, double blinding and placebo-controls—large trials fail in cancer precisely *because they are large.* These large studies were based on the assumption that cancers arising in one organ are much alike, and differ little between patients. Genomics has debunked that assumption. But that error resulted in decades of time wasted, as large studies repeatedly tested a single treatment on large numbers of cancer patients, each with essentially different diseases. An inescapable truth is that patients—and their cancers—are less alike than investigators had previously imagined.

Fortunately, the anti-bias tools of randomization, double-blinding, and placebo controls can be designed into any experiment, large or tiny, including those trials that, like mine, have an n of 1.

Research designs are rapidly being developed that allow rigorous study of the single patient, one whose condition is approached with an assortment of treatments, including medications, personalized nutrition, psychosocial interventions, supplements, and exercise.

Wondrous new tools are driving this change—genomics, epigenomics, and metabolomics to name only a few—tools that reveal what makes each of us unique. Thus the study of large, imperfectly-homogenized experimental and control groups becomes less relevant.

Advanced single-subject study designs, new technology that can access and display the myriad expressions of our biological individuality, and the ascendancy of whole-systems approaches to treatment are here to stay. And they are changing how the world practices medicine. A new clinical approach, integrative medicine, has taken on the duty of ushering into the clinic the next research paradigm, $n = 1$.

This paradigm rests however, on an old foundation, on an ancient truth, a wisdom known to all true healers, past and present. That wisdom is this: when we are ill and in need of care, we are, each of us, an n of 1. ❦

GLENN SABIN'S
ACKNOWLEDGEMENTS

MY STORY AND THIS BOOK would not have been possible without the incredible support of my amazing wife, Linda.

I am forever grateful to Dawn Lemanne, MD, MPH, who, after pushing me for some time to document my story, finally heard these words: "Dawn, I am ready to write my book—but only if you are willing to do the heavy lifting." She obliged.

My medical care A-Team: Keith I. Block, MD, the father of modern integrative oncology and my good friend; Bruce R. Kressel, MD, for his compassion and warmth, and Lee M. Nadler, MD, a brilliant, curious investigator who supported my little experiment.

My early mentors: Ross Pelton, RPh, and Irwin Rosenberg, RPh. Donald I. Abrams, MD, for making me laugh, and for nominating me to the board of Society for Integrative Oncology; Jan Adrian, for my first keynote to cancer patients; Lise Alschuler, ND, for all you do to educate cancer patients; Jorge Arciniega, JD, for having my back; Marie Beswick-Arthur, for sharpening my prose; Penny B. Block, PhD, for advocating the incredible power of A-Teams; Danielle Bouchard, Mindy Carter and Zaf Kahn, for keeping my gym in top shape; T. Colin Campbell, PhD, for sitting in the first row listening intently; Barrie R. Cassileth, MS, PhD, for creating the academic forum to openly explore the science of integrative oncology; Ellan Cates, for keeping me on message; Lorenzo Cohen, PhD, for getting funded, often, and doing the work that needs doing; Gary Deng, MD, PhD, for giving continuous encouragement; Norman Drevo and Victor Tortoro, for keeping the GTO running; Moshe Frenkel, MD, for exploring what's behind exceptional patients; Charlotte Gyllenhaal, PhD, because you are an angel; Cheri Hanson, for articulating my brand; Paul Jarvis, for making me look good; Alexander Karelis, for your eagle eye; David L. Katz, MD, for teaching that the best and often only cure is true prevention; Satkirin Khalsa, MD, for your amazing spirit and outlook; Mikhail Kogan, MD, for serving the underserved; Ruth Marlin, MD, for meditating with me before talks; Debra Mayer, JD, for being a mensch; Dwight L. McKee, MD, for your fiery intellect and support of my family; Lee Mergner, for keeping the doors open and lights on; Michele Mittelman, RN, MPH, for hanging out for bone marrow biopsies, and for your amazing grace; Simona A. Levi-Minzi, JD, PhD, for being so selfless while I was figuring things out; Matthew Mumber, MD, for my first speaking gig; Dean Ornish, MD, for your thoughtful foreword and incredible legacy; Matt Rippetoe, for capturing the cover just right; David S. Rosenthal, MD, for your early support; Jeffrey Sabin, for your unwavering backing, friendship and love; Gordon Saxe, MD, PhD, for seeing the big picture; Karen Shatzkin, JD, for keeping me safe; Bernie Siegel, MD, for the earliest inspiration; Lawrence Stern, JD, for understanding my mission and providing some leeway; Jacqueline Tschernia, for connecting me with the leading lights; John Weeks, for your early integrative mentorship and institutional vault; Jeffrey D. White, MD, for empowering investigators and being an amazing listener; Eric Wynne, for your cover vision; Kelly A. Turner, PhD, for artfully articulating and championing radical remissions; Ruth Westreich, for your brilliant mind and innate instincts in support of a better health system.

DR. LEMANNE'S
ACKNOWLEDGEMENTS

Nancy A. Noyce, MD, MPH, for cogent advice and innumerable readings; Melissa Joyce Hendricks, for generous corrections and cheerleading; Sarah Poynton, PhD, for probing with her scientific spoon a sometimes messy stew; Deborah Gordon, MD, for straightening out bent phrases.

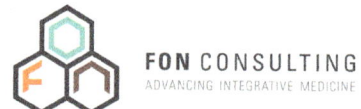
This report published in a peer-reviewed journal
discusses the technical details of Glenn's case:

Lemanne D, Block K I, Kressel B R, et al. (December 29, 2015)
A Case of Complete and Durable Molecular Remission of
Chronic Lymphocytic Leukemia Following Treatment with
Epigallocatechin-3-gallate, an Extract of Green Tea. Cureus 7(12):
e441. doi:10.7759/cureus.441

CPSIA information can be obtained
at www.ICGtesting.com
Printed in the USA
BVOW05s0344191116

468363BV00001B/1/P